QIGONG FOR HEALTH AND MARTIAL ARTS

QIGONG FOR HEALTH
AND MARTIAL ARTS

EXERCISES & MEDITATION

氣功-健康和武學上之應用

DR. YANG, JWING-MING

YMAA Publication Center
Boston, Mass. USA

YMAA Publication Center
4354 Washington Street
Boston, Massachusetts, 02131

10   9   8   7

Publisher's Cataloging in Publication
(Prepared by Quality Books Inc.)

Yang, Jwing-Ming, 1946-
    Qigong for health & martial arts : exercises and
meditation / author Jwing-Ming Yang. — 2nd ed.
    p. cm.
    Includes bibliographical references and index.
    ISBN: 1-886969-57-4

    1. Ch'i kung. 2. Ch'i kung—Therapeutic use. I.
Title.

RA781.8.Y363 1998   613.7'148
                                                QBI98-82

Figures 3-3, 3-4, 3-5, 3-6, 3-7, 3-8, 3-9, 3-12, and 3-13 modified by Sarah Noack.
Original images copyright ©1994 by TechPool Studios Corp. USA, 1463 Warrensville
Center Road, Cleveland, OH 44121.

Disclaimer:
The author and publisher of this material are NOT RESPONSIBLE in any manner
whatsoever for any injury which may occur through reading or following the
instructions in this manual.
The activities, physical or otherwise, described in this material may be too strenuous
or dangerous for some people, and the reader(s) should consult a physician before
engaging in them.

Acknowledgments

First Edition—1985

Thanks to John Gilbert Jones, Russell Steinberg, and Kenneth Silva for general help with the work. Thanks to the editor, Michael Braun, and special thanks to Alan Dougall for proofing the manuscript and contributing many valuable suggestions and discussions. Thanks to John Casagrande, Jr. for the drawings and cover design. Thanks also to Angie Adams and John Dufresne for typesetting.

Second Edition—1998

In this new edition, I would like to express many thanks to Mei-Ling Yang for general help and Ramel Rones for appearing in many of the photographs. To Milan Vigil and Doug Smith for proofing, and to Andrew Murray for editing. Special thanks to Ilana Rosenberg for the cover design, Sarah Noack for her work with the illustrations, and to Tim Comrie for the photography.

Romanization of Chinese Words

YMAA Publication Center uses the Pinyin romanization system of Chinese to English. Pinyin is standard in the People's Republic of China, and in several world organizations, including the United Nations. Pinyin, which was introduced in China in the 1950's, replaces the Wade-Giles and Yale systems.

Some common conversions:

Pinyin	Also Spelled As	Pronunciation
Qi	Chi	chē
Qigong	Chi Kung	chē kŭng
Qin Na	Chin Na	chǐn nă
Jin	Jing	jǐn
Gongfu	Kung Fu	gŏng foo
Taijiquan	Tai Chi Chuan	tǐ jē chüén

For more information, please refer to *The People's Republic of China: Administrative Atlas, The Reform of the Chinese Written Language,* or a contemporary manual of style.

Contents

About the Author

Yang, Jwing-Ming, Ph.D. 楊俊敏博士

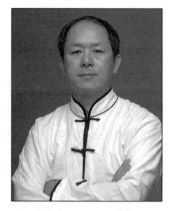

Dr. Yang, Jwing-Ming was born on August 11th, 1946, in Xinzhu Xian (新竹縣), Taiwan (台灣), Republic of China (中華民國). He started his Wushu (武術) (Gongfu or Kung Fu, 功夫) training at the age of fifteen under Shaolin White Crane (Bai He, 少林白鶴) Master Cheng, Gin-Gsao (曾金灶). Master Cheng originally learned Taizuquan (太祖拳) from his grandfather when he was a child. When Master Cheng was fifteen years old, he started learning White Crane from Master Jin, Shao-Feng (金紹峰), and followed him for twenty-three years until Master Jin's death.

In thirteen years of study (1961-1974 A.D.) under Master Cheng, Dr. Yang became an expert in the White Crane Style of Chinese martial arts, which includes both the use of barehands and of various weapons such as saber, staff, spear, trident, two short rods, and many other weapons. With the same master he also studied White Crane Qigong (氣功), Qin Na (or Chin Na, 擒拿), Tui Na (推拿) and Dian Xue massages (點穴按摩), and herbal treatment.

At the age of sixteen, Dr. Yang began the study of Yang Style Taijiquan (楊氏太極拳) under Master Kao Tao (高濤). After learning from Master Kao, Dr. Yang continued his study and research of Taijiquan in Taipei (台北) with several masters and senior practitioners such as Master Li, Mao-Ching (李茂清) and Mr. Wilson Chen (陳威伸). Master Li learned his Taijiquan from the well-known Master Han, Ching-Tang (韓慶堂), and Mr. Chen learned his Taijiquan from Master Zhang, Xiang-San (張祥三). Dr. Yang has mastered the Taiji barehand sequence, pushing hands, the two-man fighting sequence, Taiji sword, Taiji saber, and Taiji Qigong.

When Dr. Yang was eighteen years old he entered Tamkang College (淡江學院) in Taipei Xian to study Physics. In college he began the study of traditional Shaolin Long Fist (Changquan or Chang Chuan, 少林長拳) with Master Li, Mao-Ching at the Tamkang College Guoshu Club (淡江國術社)(1964-1968 A.D.), and eventually became an assistant instructor under Master Li. In 1971, he completed his M.S. degree in Physics at the National Taiwan University (台灣大學), and then served in the Chinese Air Force from 1971 to 1972. In the service, Dr. Yang taught Physics at the Junior Academy of the Chinese Air Force (空軍幼校) while also teaching Wushu. After being honorably discharged in 1972, he returned to Tamkang College to teach Physics and resumed study under Master Li, Mao-Ching. From Master Li, Dr. Yang learned Northern Style

Wushu, which includes both barehand (especially kicking) techniques and numerous weapons.

In 1974, Dr. Yang came to the United States to study Mechanical Engineering at Purdue University. At the request of a few students, Dr. Yang began to teach Gongfu (Kung Fu), which resulted in the foundation of the Purdue University Chinese Kung Fu Research Club in the spring of 1975. While at Purdue, Dr. Yang also taught college-credited courses in Taijiquan. In May of 1978, he was awarded a Ph.D. in Mechanical Engineering by Purdue.

In 1980, Dr. Yang moved to Houston to work for Texas Instruments. While in Houston, he founded Yang's Shaolin Kung Fu Academy, which was eventually taken over by his disciple, Mr. Jeffery Bolt, after Dr. Yang moved to Boston in 1982. Dr. Yang founded Yang's Martial Arts Academy (YMAA) in Boston on October 1, 1982.

In January of 1984, he gave up his engineering career to devote more time to research, writing, and teaching. In March of 1986, he purchased property in the Jamaica Plain area of Boston to be used as the headquarters of the new organization, Yang's Martial Arts Association. The organization has continued to expand, and, on July 1st 1989, YMAA became just one division of Yang's Oriental Arts Association, Inc. (YOAA, Inc.).

In summary, Dr. Yang has been involved in Chinese Wushu since 1961. During this time, he has spent thirteen years learning Shaolin White Crane (Bai He), Shaolin Long Fist (Changquan), and Taijiquan. Dr. Yang has more than twenty-eight years of instructional experience: seven years in Taiwan, five years at Purdue University, two years in Houston, Texas, and fourteen years in Boston, Massachusetts.

In addition, Dr. Yang has been invited to offer seminars around the world to share his knowledge of Chinese martial arts and Qigong. The countries he has visited include Canada, Mexico, France, Italy, Poland, England, Ireland, Portugal, Switzerland, Germany, Hungary, Spain, Holland, Latvia, South Africa, and Saudi Arabia.

Since 1986, YMAA has become an international organization, and currently has thirty schools in the following countries: Poland, Portugal, France, Italy, Holland, Hungary, South Africa, the United Kingdom, Canada, and the United States. Many of Dr. Yang's books and videotapes have been translated into French, Italian, Spanish, Polish, Czech, Bulgarian, Russian, and Hungarian.

Dr. Yang has published twenty-one other volumes on the martial arts and Qigong:

1. *Shaolin Chin Na;* Unique Publications, Inc., 1980.

2. *Shaolin Long Fist Kung Fu;* Unique Publications, Inc., 1981.

3. *Yang Style Tai Chi Chuan;* Unique Publications, Inc., 1981.

4. *Introduction to Ancient Chinese Weapons;* Unique Publications, Inc., 1985

5. *Qigong for Health & Martial Arts;* YMAA Publication Center, 1985.

6. *Northern Shaolin Sword;* YMAA Publication Center, 1985.

7. *Tai Chi Theory and Martial Power;* YMAA Publication Center, 1986.

8. *Tai Chi Chuan Martial Applications,* YMAA Publication Center, 1986.

9. *Analysis of Shaolin Chin Na;* YMAA Publication Center, 1987.

10. *Eight Simple Qigong Exercises for Health;* YMAA Publication Center, 1988.

11. *The Root of Chinese Qigong—Secrets for Health, Longevity, & Enlightenment* ; YMAA Publication Center, 1989.

12. *Muscle/Tendon Changing and Marrow/Brain Washing Chi Kung—The Secret of Youth;* YMAA Publication Center, 1989.

13. *Hsing Yi Chuan—Theory and Applications;* YMAA Publication Center, 1990.

14. *The Essence of Tai Chi Chi Kung—Health and Martial Arts;* YMAA Publication Center, 1990.

15. *Arthritis—The Chinese Way of Healing & Prevention;* YMAA Publication Center, 1991.

16. *Chinese Qigong Massage—General Massage;* YMAA Publication Center, 1992.

17. *How to Defend Yourself;* YMAA Publication Center, 1992.

18. *Baguazhang—Emei Baguazhang;* YMAA Publication Center, 1994.

19. *Comprehensive Applications of Shaolin Chin Na—The Practical Defense of Chinese Seizing Arts;* YMAA Publication Center, 1995.

20. *Taiji Chin Na—The Seizing Art of Taijiquan;* YMAA Publication Center, 1995.

21. *The Essence of Shaolin White Crane;* YMAA Publication Center, 1996.

22. *Back Pain—Chinese Qigong for Healing and Prevention;* YMAA Publication Center, 1997.

Dr. Yang has also produced the following videotapes:

1. *Yang Style Tai Chi Chuan and Its Applications;* YMAA Publication Center, 1984.

2. *Shaolin Long Fist Kung Fu—Lien Bu Chuan and Its Applications;* YMAA Publication Center, 1985.

3. *Shaolin Long Fist Kung Fu—Gung Li Chuan and Its Applications;* YMAA Publication Center, 1986.

4. *Analysis of Shaolin Chin Na;* YMAA Publication Center, 1987.

5. *Eight Simple Qigong Exercises for Health—The Eight Pieces of Brocade;* YMAA Publication Center, 1987.

6. *Chi Kung for Tai Chi Chuan;* YMAA Publication Center, 1990.

7. *Arthritis—The Chinese Way of Healing and Prevention;* YMAA Publication Center, 1991.

8. *Qigong Massage—Self Massage;* YMAA Publication Center, 1992.

9. *Qigong Massage—With a Partner;* YMAA Publication Center, 1992.

10. *Defend Yourself 1—Unarmed Attack;* YMAA Publication Center, 1992.

11. *Defend Yourself 2—Knife Attack;* YMAA Publication Center, 1992.

12. *Comprehensive Applications of Shaolin Chin Na 1;* YMAA Publication Center, 1995.

13. *Comprehensive Applications of Shaolin Chin Na 2;* YMAA Publication Center, 1995.

14. *Shaolin Long Fist Kung Fu—Yi Lu Mai Fu & Er Lu Mai Fu;* YMAA Publication Center, 1995.

15. *Shaolin Long Fist Kung Fu—Shi Zi Tang;* YMAA Publication Center, 1995.

16. *Taiji Chin Na;* YMAA Publication Center, 1995.

17. *Emei Baguazhang—1; Basic Training, Qigong, Eight Palms, and Applications;* YMAA Publication Center, 1995.

18. *Emei Baguazhang—2; Swimming Body Baguazhang and Its Applications;* YMAA Publication Center, 1995.

19. *Emei Baguazhang—3; Bagua Deer Hook Sword and Its Applications;* YMAA Publication Center, 1995.

20. *Xingyiquan—12 Animal Patterns and Their Applications;* YMAA Publication Center, 1995.

21. *24 and 48 Simplified Taijiquan;* YMAA Publication Center, 1995.

22. *White Crane Hard Qigong;* YMAA Publication Center, 1997.

23. *White Crane Soft Qigong;* YMAA Publication Center, 1997.

24. *Xiao Hu Yan—Intermediate Level Long Fist Sequence;* YMAA Publication Center, 1997.

25. *Back Pain—Chinese Qigong for Healing and Prevention;* YMAA Publication Center, 1997.

Foreword

Qigong and martial arts training are closely related. Anyone who studies martial arts should study Qigong, because without a good healthy body, how can you consider self defense?

In the past in China, there were no Western sports like football, basketball, swimming, or running. If parents wanted their children to be healthy and do some physical exercise, martial arts training was one of the only ways. However, martial arts training is not just training for fighting. The first step is to train the person to be healthy, through internal training. This training deals with the Qi and is very different from Western exercises, which are only physical and external.

The concept of Qi is at the foundation of all Chinese cultural skills. Every kind of skill is related to Qi. When a person says you have good Qi, it could mean your spirit, your energy, or that you are strong and healthy. But if they say your Qi has gone, then so has your spirit and energy and your body will be weak and tired. Therefore, Qi is very important.

Dr. Yang, Jwing-Ming has an enormous amount of knowledge of Western science and Chinese cultural skills. He is famous throughout the Qigong and martial arts world. Anybody who seriously studies martial arts or Qigong has heard his name, seen his articles, or read his books.

For many years he has worked hard to promote Chinese martial arts and Qigong and brought his vast knowledge and experience of traditional Chinese skills to the West. He has a lot to offer, and it is very good to see this book in its second edition. This is an excellent opportunity for readers to benefit a great deal.

Michael Tse

Born in Hong Kong, Michael Tse has spent the last twenty years training with some of the most famous teachers in Hong Kong and China, including the famous Dayan Qigong master Yang Meijun, and Yip Chun, the eldest son of Yip Man. He also the director of the Tse Qigong Center in the United Kingdom, and publisher of the UK's Qi Magazine.

Preface

First Edition

"Gongfu" (Kung Fu, 功夫) in Chinese means an achievement or activity that requires time, energy, and patience. Qigong (Chi Kung, 氣功)(pronounced chee goong) means the Gongfu of internal energy circulation. Qi (氣) has been known for more than a decade by the Western world, but it remains a mysterious concept to most Westerners, and even to many Qigong practitioners. Many people have experienced health benefits from Qigong, although very few of them really understand the principles or theory behind it, the relationship between Qigong and acupuncture, or the connection between Qigong and the martial arts. The author hopes that this volume, which specializes in Qigong, will help to dispel the mystery and thus benefit more people.

In this book, the first chapter will explain the general concept of Qigong, its history, and its relationship to health and the martial arts. The second chapter will introduce Wai Dan (external elixir, 外丹) techniques to promote external/internal local Qi circulation. The history of the creator of Shaolin Wai Dan, Da Mo (達磨), and the book he wrote on the subject, the *Yi Jin Jing* (易筋經), will also be discussed. The third chapter will present primary Qigong training called Nei Dan (internal elixir, 內丹), or internal/internal Dan Tian Qi (丹田氣) circulation, which was developed by the Daoists and Buddhists. The fourth chapter will explain the use of Qigong to improve and maintain health. And finally, the fifth chapter will discuss in general the application of Qigong to the martial arts. An additional volume will be necessary to cover the principles and methods of training in detail. The author hopes to be able to do this in the near future. Those who wish further information are referred to the author's books *Yang Style Tai Chi Chuan* for specifics on that system, and to *Shaolin Chin Na* for information on cavity press.

Dr. Yang, Jwing-Ming
Boston, 1985

Second Edition

Since the first edition of this book was published in 1985, more than thirty-five thousand copies have been sold. This surprised me, because the concept of Qigong is still new to most Westerners. The concept of Chinese Qigong was first introduced to America through acupuncture, when President Nixon visited mainland China in 1973. Nixon's visit accelerated the cultural exchange between the East and the West, and one of the goals of this exchange is the promotion of world harmony through mutual understanding.

During this exciting era, the mission of my life has been to translate traditional Chinese documents into English to expedite this cultural exchange. In addition to translating these documents, I also include my thirty-five years of personal experience in Qigong. This book was my first of this effort.

This book contains basic, fundamental information which is very useful for Qigong beginners. In addition, to those martial artists who are interested in knowing about the internal side of martial arts training, this book can be considered a key to the entrance of the martial arts Qigong garden. Since 1985, I have written other Qigong and Chinese martial arts books. Many are related to Qigong for health, longevity, and spiritual enlightenment. These are:

- *Eight Simple Qigong Exercises for Health*
- *The Root of Chinese Qigong—Secrets for Health, Longevity, & Enlightenment*
- *Muscle/Tendon Changing and Marrow/Brain Washing Chi Kung—The Secret of Youth*
- *The Essence of Taiji Qigong—The Internal Foundation of Taijiquan*
- *Arthritis—The Chinese Way of Healing & Prevention*
- *Chinese Qigong Massage—General Massage*
- *The Essence of Shaolin White Crane*
- *Back Pain—Chinese Qigong for Healing and Prevention*

After reading this book, if you are interested in further exploring this Qigong garden, you should not hesitate to read the above books. For health and healing Qigong exercises, videotapes are also available. The books and the videotapes are an easy way to learn self-healing. Today, Qigong is recognized as one of the most effective alternative (or complimentary) medicines. I believe that Qigong will become the major force in prevention and healing in the next two decades.

In the new edition of this book, a few changes have been made. First, all the Chinese has been changed to Pinyin, which is now the most popular romanization system in Western society. Second, portions of the content have been updated. Third, the typesetting has been improved to make the book easier to read, and new photographs have replaced the old. Finally, a glossary of Chinese terms and an index have been included.

I hope this book will lead you to further Qigong study and practice. I also hope that all qualified Qigong teachers and researchers will share their understanding and experience with open, scientific and logical minds. Only then can we expect to see the bright future of Qigong study and development.

Dr. Yang, Jwing-Ming
Boston, 1997

Chapter 1
Introduction

介紹

1-1. General Introduction

Qigong (氣功), also called Nei Gong (Internal Gongfu, 內功), is a practice that has been used by the Chinese people for thousands of years—both to improve and maintain their health and to develop greater power for the martial arts. Gong (功) means work in Chinese, and Qi (氣) is the energy that circulates within the body, so Qigong means the cultivation of the body's energy to increase and control its circulation.

Although it has been widely practiced for a very long time, many people are confused about Qigong, even in China, and many doubt the possibility of internal energy development, or even the existence of Qi. There are several reasons for this:

1. Until as recently as fifty years ago, most Qigong experts would only teach family members or trusted students, so Qigong knowledge was not widespread.

2. Many of the techniques were developed and cultivated by Buddhist or Daoist monks who would not spread their teachings outside their own temples.

3. Because most people were ignorant of Qigong, it was superstitiously regarded as magic.

4. Lastly, some people learned incorrect methods and experienced no effects from the training, or even injured themselves. This resulted in people either being scornful or fearful of Qigong.

You should understand that Qigong has a scientific foundation and theory. It is part of the body of Chinese medicine with a history that goes back thousands of years. The most important books describing Qi and its actions are the *Qi Hua Lun (Theory of Qi Variations,* 氣化論), which explains the relationship between Qi and nature, and the *Jing Luo Lun (Theory of Qi Channels and Branches,* 經絡論), which describes Qi circulation throughout the human body. ("Jing," 經 means primary Qi channel or meridian. "Luo," 絡 refers to the subchannels that branch out from them). A channel, or meridian, is a major connector of the internal organs with the rest of the body. These channels frequently are co-located with major nerves or arteries, but the correspondence is not complete, and it seems that they are neither nerves nor blood vessels, but simply the main routes for Qi. There are twelve main channels and two major vessels (Mai, 脈) in the body. Along these channels are found the "cavities" (Xue, 穴), sometimes known as acupuncture points, which can be used to stimulate the entire Qi system.

Qigong is also based upon the theory of Yin (陰) and Yang (陽), which describes the relationship of complementary qualities such as soft and hard, female and male, dark and light, or slow and fast. According to Yin/Yang theory, nature strives for harmony, so that all things are neutral or balanced. Since people are part of nature, they should also strive for balance.

Included in Yin/Yang theory is the theory of the five elements or phases. The five elements are Jin (metal, 金), Mu (wood, 木), Shui (water, 水), Huo (fire, 火), and Tu (earth, 土). These elements are somewhat different from the old European elements of fire, air, water, earth. Again, because people are part of nature, they participate in and are affected by the interplay of the elements.

According to Chinese medicine, there are two ways to study health and illness. The first way is externally, called "Wai Xiang Jie Pou" (外象解剖). The second is internally, called "Nei Shi Gongfu" (內視功夫). Wai Xiang Jie Pou is a way to understand the human body by dissection or by acting physically on the body and observing the results, as in modern laboratory experiments. In Nei Shi Gongfu the researcher learns by introspection. He observes his own body and sensations and develops medical knowledge this way.

The Western world has specialized almost exclusively in Wai Xiang (外象) and has viewed Nei Shi (內視) as "unscientific," although in recent years this attitude has been changing among the general populace, if not within the medical profession.

Nei Shi Gongfu developed from observations of the correspondence between changes in nature and the way people felt, and the discovery of Qi variations. "Nature" here includes periodic cycles (Tian Shi, 天時) such as time of day, the seasons, air pressure, wind direction, and humidity. It also includes geographical features (Di Li, 地理) such as altitude, distance from the equator, and distance from large bodies of water, such as an ocean or a lake. These empirical observations led to the conclusion that Qi circulation is related to nature, and led to a search for ways for people to harmonize with natural variations.

In addition, Qi was also observed to be closely related to human affairs (Ren Shi, 人事). This includes the relationship of Qi to sound, emotion, and food. Because Qi flow is controlled by the brain, agitation of the brain by emotion will affect Qi circulation. The sounds people made in various situations were also observed. For example, in cold weather the sound "Si" (嘶) is used in combination with breathing deeply and keeping the limbs close to the body to help keep warm. The pain from cuts can be relieved by making the sound "Xu" (嘘) and blowing air into the cut. The "Xu" sound helps to stop the bleeding and calm the liver, and the relaxation of this organ in turn relieves the pain. The sound "Hei" (嘿)is used to increase a person's working strength. The sound "Ha" (哈) will help to relieve fevers the same way a dog's panting helps it to bear the heat. From all these observations it was concluded that different sounds can relieve the pressure or strain on different organs, and since inner organs were related to the channels, the Qi circulation was affected as well.

The relationship of Qi and food is illustrated by the fact that drinking too much alcohol or eating too much deep fried food will strain the liver and thus affect the Qi circulation in the liver channel.

After a long period of observation people began to understand that Qi circulation affected their health, and they began to investigate ways to improve this circulation. Methods were found and forms were created that proved effective, and this was the beginning of Qigong.

1-2. Historical Survey of Chinese Qigong

There are four major divisions or schools of Qigong practice and theory that have been developed by four groups: the Confucians, the Physicians, the Buddhist and Daoist monks, and the Chinese martial artists. These groups are not mutually exclusive. For example, a physician studying the workings of Qi might also be a Confucian or Daoist. However, the works we have are usually identifiable as belonging to one particular group.

The Confucians were primarily interested in the workings of human society rather than in withdrawal and self perfection. For them, the purpose of Qigong was to make people more fit to fulfill their function. This group includes many famous artists and scholars, and they frequently expressed their views on Qigong in poetry. The most famous of these poets are Li Bai (李白), Su, Dong-Po (蘇東坡), and Bai, Ju-Yi (白居易). Su, Dong-Po was the co-author with Shen, Cun-Zhong (沈存中) of *Su Shen Lian Fang* (*Good Prescriptions of Su and Shen*, 蘇沈良方).

The physicians were not specifically aligned with any philosophical group, although their work often has recognizable Daoist influences. Their work is distinguished by its emphasis on the balance of Qi.

The Buddhist monks emphasized becoming free from the suffering of existence through awareness. Their primary method was still meditation with the use of breathing directed toward stilling the mind. Although considerable Qi circulation was developed, it was not the primary goal. The Daoists are associated with withdrawal from society to perfect the self and achieve immortality. To do this they used Qigong and alchemy, and these two methods are frequently discussed together. In fact two terms used in this book, Wai Dan (外丹) and Nei Dan (內丹), which describe methods of improving Qi circulation, originally meant the alchemical elixir of immortality.

The Chinese martial artists made many contributions to the field of Qigong. Generally, their

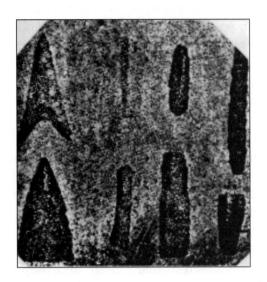

Figure 1-1. Bian Shi Found at Henan Province.

use of Qigong focuses on strength and power development, body protection, health maintenance, and the treatment of injury. Martial Qigong will be explored in greater detail throughout this book.

Historical records from before the Han dynasty (漢朝) are very fragmented and much of the history of the period is conjecture. Traditionally, the history of Qi theory begins with the birth of Chinese medicine in the reign of the Yellow Emperor, Huang Di (2697-2597 B.C., 黃帝). The book that is the theoretical foundation for Chinese medicine to the present day, the *Nei Jing Su Wen, (Classic on Internal Medicine,* 內經素問), is attributed to Huang Di, but modern scholars now believe it to be a work of the Han dynasty.

The *Yi Jing,* (易經), on the other hand, is a very old book, believed to date before 2400 B.C. It discusses all the variations of nature in a compact form. Natural forces are represented by the eight trigrams, and these are combined into sixty-four hexagrams. These figures have permeated every aspect of Chinese culture, so it is not surprising that the eight trigrams are used to describe the circulation of Qi in the body.

By the time of the Shang dynasty (1766-1122 B.C., 商朝) people used stone probes called Bian Shi (砭石) (Figure 1-1) to stimulate cavities on the channels which affected the Qi circulation and relieved pain. They had already discovered that a sharp instrument was better than just fingers for stimulating pressure points.

In the sixth century B.C. the philosopher Lao Zi (老子)(or Li Er, 李耳) described breathing techniques for increasing the life span in his classic, the *Dao De Jing* (*Classic on the Virtue of the Dao,* 道德經)(especially chapter 10). This was the first record of the use of breathing techniques to increase Qi circulation and thus increase the length of life.

The *Shi Ji* (*Historical Record,* 史紀) shows that by the Spring and Autumn and Warring States periods (722-222 B.C., 春秋戰國) more complete methods of breath training had evolved.

Around 300 B.C., the Daoist philosopher Zhuang Zi (莊子) described the relationship between breathing and health in his book *Nan Hua Jing* (南華經). It states: "The real person's (i.e., immortal's) breathing reaches down to their heels. The normal person's breathing in the throat."[1] This confirms that a breathing method of Qi circulation was being used by some Daoists at that time.

During the Qin and Han dynasties (255 B.C. to 220 A.D., 秦漢) several books related to Qigong were written. The *Nan Jing* (*Classic on Disorders,* 難經) by the famous doctor Bian Que (扁鵲) describes the use of breathing to increase Qi circulation. The *Han Shu Yi Wen Zhi* (*Han's Book of Arts and Scholarship,* 漢書藝文志) describes four methods of Qigong training. The *Jin Kui Yao Lue* (*Prescriptions from the Golden Chamber,* 金匱要略) by Zhang, Zhong-Jing (張仲景) describes the use of breathing and acupuncture to maintain good Qi flow. The *Zhou Yi Can Tong Qi* (*A Comparative Study of the Zhou (dynasty) Book of Changes,* 周易參同契) by Wei, Bo-Yang (魏伯陽) describes the relationship between humans and natural forces and with Qi. Also during this time, anatomical knowledge grew through the dissection of bodies. The structure of the human body in relation to the channel and nervous systems was better understood, and the existence of Qi circulation gained wider acceptance.

During the Western Jin dynasty (265-317 A.D., 西晉), the famous physician Hua Tuo (華陀) used acupuncture for anesthesia in surgery. In addition, he spread the Daoist Jun Qing (君倩) method, which imitated the five animals—tiger, deer, monkey, bear, and bird—to generate local Qi circulation. This is a form of Wai Dan Qigong and is called Wu Qin Xi (Five Animal Sport, 五禽戲). The physician Ge Hong (葛洪) mentions using the mind to guide and increase the flow of Qi in his book *Bao Po Zi* (*Embrace the Simplicity,* 抱朴子).

Sometime between 420 and 581 A.D. Tao, Hong-Jing (陶弘景) compiled the *Yang Shen Yen Ming Lu* (*Records of Nourishing the Body and Extending Life,* 養身延命錄) which records many Qigong techniques for improving health.

During the Liang dynasty (502-557 A.D., 梁朝), Da Mo (達磨), a Buddhist monk from India, arrived at the Shaolin temple (少林寺)(see chapter 2 for Da

Mo's history). Da Mo saw that the monks were weak and could do very little, and he was so disturbed by this that he shut himself away to ponder the problem. He stayed in seclusion for nine years. When he emerged he had written two books: *Yi Jin Jing (Muscle/Tendon Changing Classic,* 易筋經) and *Xi Sui Jing (Brain/Marrow Washing Classic,* 洗髓經). *The Muscle/Tendon Changing Classic* taught the priests how to regain their health and change their physical bodies from weak to strong. The *Marrow/Brain Washing Classic* taught the priests how to use Qi to clean the bone marrow and strengthen the blood and the immune system, as well as how to energize the brain and attain enlightenment. Because the *Marrow/Brain Washing Classic* was harder to understand and practice, the training methods were passed down in secret to only a very few disciples in each generation.

The exercises in the *Muscle/Tendon Changing Classic* are a form of Wai Dan (external-internal Qigong, 外丹氣功) using concentration to develop local Qi and increase Qi circulation. The monks practiced these methods and found that their physical strength and power greatly increased. This training was integrated into martial arts forms practiced at the temple, and became the first known application of Qigong to the martial arts.

The Shaolin priests continued developing these Qigong methods and combined them with five sets of fighting forms that imitate the movements of animals known for their fighting ability. These were the tiger, the leopard, the dragon, the snake, and the crane. These animal names are still found in Gongfu styles. Five animal martial training is called Shaolin Five Animal Fists (Shaolin Wu Xing Quan, 少林五形拳).

The development of Qigong methods and theory continued during the Sui and Tang dynasties (589-907 A.D., 隋、唐). Chao, Yuan-Fang (巢元方) compiled the *Zhu Bing Yuan Hou Lun (Thesis on the Origins and Symptoms of Various Diseases,* 諸病源候論), which is a veritable encyclopedia of methods. He lists 260 different ways of increasing the flow of Qi. The *Qian Jin Fang (Thousand Gold Prescriptions,* 千金方) by Sun, Si-Miao (孫思邈) describes a method of guiding Qi, introduces the use of the six sounds (see chapter 4) and their relationship with the internal organs, and also introduces a collection of massage techniques called Lao Zi's Forty-Nine Massage Techniques. *Wai Tai Mi Yao (The Extra Important Secret,* 外台密要) by Wang Tao (王濤) discusses the use of breathing and herbal therapies for Qi circulation disorders.

Between 960 and 1368 A.D. (the Song, Jin, and Yuan dynasties, 宋、金、元), several works of interest were written. *Yang Shen Jue (Life Nourishing Secrets,* 養身訣) by Zhang, An-Dao (張安道) discusses Qigong practice. *Ru Men Shi Shi (The Confucian Point of View,* 儒門視事) by Zhang, Zi-He (張子和) discusses the use of Qigong to cure external injuries such as cuts and sprains. *Lan Shi Mi Cang (Secret Library of the Orchid Room,* 蘭室密藏) by Li Guo (李果) describes Qigong and herbal remedies for internal disorders. *Ge Zhi Yu Lun (A Further Thesis of Complete Study,* 格致餘論) by Zhu, Dan-Xi (朱丹溪) provides a theoretical explanation for the use of Qigong in curing sickness.

It is during the Song dynasty (960-1280 A.D., 宋朝) that Zhang, San-Feng (張三豐) is reputed to have created Taijiquan (太極拳) at Wudang Mountain (武當). Taijiquan is a martial form of Nei Dan Qigong (內丹氣功) which builds the energy from the Dan Tian (丹田), a spot in the lower abdomen one and a half inches below the navel. Taijiquan makes use of Small Circulation (Xiao Zhou Tian, 小周天) Qigong and Grand

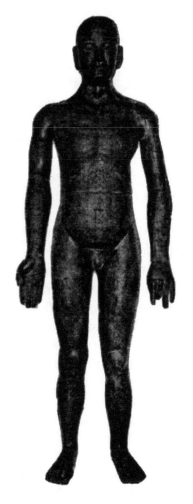

Figure 1-2. "Brass Man" by Wang, Wei-Yi

Circulation Qigong, and then applies this energy to martial uses. Small and Grand Circulation will be discussed in chapter 3 of this book.

In 1026 A.D. the famous Brass Man (a hollow brass dummy with the Qi channels and cavity locations marked on it, see Figure 1-2) was built by Wang, Wei-Yi (王唯一). This great accomplishment helped to organize acupuncture theory more systematically.

From then until the Qing dynasty (1644-1912 A.D., 清朝) the existence of Qi, its benefits to health, and its usefulness to the martial arts continued to gain acceptance among the Chinese people. Many ways of increasing Qi circulation were developed and practiced. For example Marshal Yue Fei (岳飛) who lived in the Southern Song dynasty (1127-1280 A.D., 南宋) is reputed to have been the creator of many Qigong styles. It is said that Marshal Yue Fei, seeing that his soldiers were weak, used the Da Mo's Yi Jin Jing exercises as a foundation and modified it into Shi Er Duan Jin (十二段錦) or Twelve Pieces of Brocade (later simplified into Ba Duan Jin, 八段錦 or Eight Pieces of Brocade) to train his soldiers.

Several other Qigong styles were created during this period that are still used today. The martial artists of the Emei division, located at Emei Mountain in Sichuan Province (四川省峨嵋山), still use their Hu Bu Gong (Tiger Step Gong, 虎步功) and Shi Er Zhuang (Twelve Postures, 十二庄). Another style rarely used today, but in use before the revolution is Jiao Fa Gong (Beggar Gong, 叫化功) which was practiced by beggars to enable them to withstand a life filled with exposure to the elements and irregular meals. However, this style has nearly died out.

The publication of written works on Qigong continued during the Ming and Qing dynasties (1368-1912 A.D., 明、清). *Qi Jing Ba Mai Kao (The Verifications of the Strange Channels and the Eight Vessels,* 奇經八脈考) by Li, Shi-Zhen (李時珍) discusses the relationship of Qigong with the Qi channels. *Bao Shen Bi Yao (The Secret Important Document of Body Protection,* 保身秘要) by Cao, Yuan-Bai (曹元白) examines moving and stationary Qigong. *Yang Shen Fu Yu (Brief Introduction to Nourishing the Body,* 養身膚語) by Chen, Ji-Ru (陳繼儒) discusses the three treasures of the body: Jing (essence, 精), Qi (internal energy, 氣) and Shen (spirit, 神) and how to protect and preserve these treasures. For example, both excessive retention of sperm and excessive dispersion are bad for health, so a man's sex life must be carefully regulated according to his constitution and age. *Yi Fang Ji Jie (The Total Introduction to Medical Prescriptions,* 醫方集介) by Wang, Fan-An (汪汎庵) is a review and summary of previously published material. Wang, Zu-Yuan's (王祖源) *Nei Gong Tu Shuo (Illustrated Explanation of Nei Gong,* 内功圖説) presents the Twelve Pieces of Brocade exercise, and explains the idea of using both moving and stationary Qigong.

The well known martial art Baguazhang (Eight Trigrams Palm, 八卦掌) was created during the Qing dynasty (1644-1912 A.D., 清朝) and is still practiced today. Another popular style, called Huo Long Gong (Fire Dragon Gong, 火龍功), was created toward the end of the Ming dynasty (c. 1640 A.D., 明朝) by the Taiyang (太陽) division, and is occasionally used for health purposes. Many other styles or methods have been used, but most have died out, or are known to only a few practitioners.

Since 1912 so many books have been written in China that your best resource is a good bookstore. The Qigong styles most widely known today are Taijiquan, Baguazhang, Xingyiquan, and Liu He Ba Fa, which are essentially martial arts, and Shi Er Duan Jin, Ba Duan Jin, Yi Jin Jing, and Wu Qin Xi, which are strictly health exercises.

1-3. General Principles of Chinese Qigong

In order to understand Qigong, you must understand several concepts. The first of these is Qi. Qi is the foundation of all Chinese medical theory and Qigong. It corresponds to the Greek "pneuma" and the Sanskrit "prana," and is considered to be the vital force and energy flow in all living things. According to the experience of Qigong practitioners, Qi can be best explained as a type of energy very much like electricity, which flows through the human or animal body. When this circulation becomes stagnant or stops, the person or animal will become ill or die.

Although there is no precise Western definition of Qi, it is often referred to as bioelectricity. In fact, it was recognized in the last decade that Qi is actually the bioelectricity circulating in all living things.[2 & 3]

Qi can also be explained as a medium of sensing or feeling. For example, when a person's arm is hurt, the Qi flow in the nerves of the arm is disturbed and stimulated to a higher energy state. This higher energy states causes a sensational feeling that is interpreted as pain by the brain. In addition, the difference in energy potential causes an increased flow of Qi and blood to that area to begin repairing damage. Therefore, Qi, the nervous system, the Qi channels, and the brain are intimately related to each other and can not be separated.

The second concept you should know is that of Qi channels, which circulate Qi throughout the body. For the most part the main Qi channels are found with the arteries and nerves. A glance into any anatomy book shows that large sheathes of nerve fibers accompany the arteries throughout the body. The Qi channels do also. Like arteries and nerves, the Qi channels are protected by the body's musculature, so that they are hard to affect directly. There is one spot on the body where a channel is very exposed, and that is the funny bone. This spot is called Shaohai (少海) in acupuncture and belongs to the Hand Shaoyin Heart Channel (手少陰心經). Here the channel and median nerve systems coincide. A light tap to this spot will numb the entire forearm, which demonstrates the extreme sensitivity of the channels, as well as the control they exert throughout the body.

According to Chinese medicine, there are twelve primary Qi channels (which are thought of as Qi rivers) and eight major vessels (which are thought of as Qi reservoirs) in the human body. The twelve channels (actually pairs of channels, one on either side of the body) are related to different internal organs. When the Qi is stagnant in one channel, the corresponding organ will be

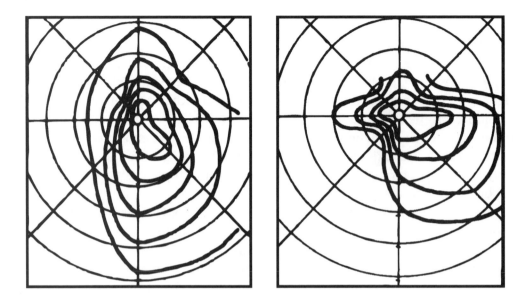

Figure 1-3. Electrical Conductivity Maps of the Skin Surface over Acupuncture Points

disordered. One of the major techniques of acupuncture is to stimulate the channel with a needle. This increases or decreases the circulation of Qi, and helps bring the malfunctioning organ back into balance.

Among the eight vessels, two are considered the most important in Chinese medicine. These two major vessels are the Ren Mai (任脈) or Conception Vessel, which runs down the front center of the body, and the Du Mai (督脈) or Governing Vessel, which runs down the center of the back and the head.

The third concept you should understand is that of acupuncture points, which are also called cavities (Xue, 穴). Along each of the channels (as well as elsewhere on the body) are points where the electrical conductivity is higher than surrounding area (Figure 1-3)[3]. These points, which are called cavities because they can often be felt as small depressions or concavities, are more sensitive than other parts of the body. These are the locations used for acupuncture, and they are also points of attack in the martial arts. Acupuncture recognizes more than seven hundred cavities, although only 108 cavities are used by martial artists. The application of power to one of the 108 cavities can result in pain, numbness of some part of the body, damage to one of the body's internal organs, unconsciousness, or even death. Of these 108 cavities, thirty-six are death cavities. That is, a strike to one of these thirty-six cavities can damage an internal organ, causing death. For example, a strike to the Jiquan cavity (H-1)(極泉) on the heart channel found in the armpit, can shock the heart so severely that it goes into fatal spasms. The seventy-two remaining cavities are not death cavities, but striking them can cause numbness or unconsciousness, provided exactly the right spot is hit at the right time.

The fourth concept you should know is that the circulation of Qi is governed by the time of day and the season of the year. Qi circulates within the body from conception to death, but the part of the body where the Qi is the strongest changes around the clock. However, Qi circulates continuously within the two major vessels without being affected by time. Because of the variability of Qi circulation, you must be knowledgeable about it to use Qigong effectively.

The most important thing to remember is that everything is controlled by the mind. Western science has proven that we use only thirty to forty percent of our brain capacity. If a person could be trained to use more than this amount, he or she would be a genius. Science believes that this can be done through meditation and concentration training. It is well documented that a hypnotized person can do things that are far beyond what is possible when in a normal state. Meditation is a form of self-hypnosis that can lead you toward this sort of increased performance.

In Qigong training the mind controls the flow of Qi, just as it controls other body functions. You may have experienced ways in which the mind causes reactions in your body. Thinking about frightening things can make you sweat. Thinking of a tense situation can cause you to tighten your muscles so much that your whole body becomes sore. In this case your mind caused a chemical reaction, i.e. the generation of acid in your tight muscles. Your mind can also relax your body just by thinking about it. Many people are using this approach to control their pulse or blood pressure without drugs.

In Qigong training, concentration is the key to success. By concentrating attention on the abdomen and doing certain exercises, Qi is generated and circulated throughout the body. This leads to the development of extra energy and its more efficient use; for example, allowing a martial artist to strike with tremendous power and to resist the penetration of an opponent's power into his or her body. The amount of Qi that can be generated is determined largely by the level of concentration.

There are several common ways to raise Qi to a higher energy state. The first way is called Wai Dan (外丹). In this method, Qi is stimulated at a particular location in the body by continued muscular exertion combined with concentration. For example, if you hold your arms extended in one position for several minutes, the shoulders will become very warm from the Qi accumulation. When you relax your shoulders, this higher energy will flow to places with a lower energy state. Wai Dan exercises have been used in China for many centuries. Wai Dan was later coordinated with martial techniques by the Shaolin monks. Chapter 2 will explain this method in detail.

The second way of increasing Qi circulation is called Nei Dan (內丹). In this method Qi is accumulated at the Dan Tian, a spot an inch and a half below the navel. Once sufficient Qi has accumulated, then you use your mind to guide the Qi to circulate in the two major vessels—the Governing Vessel and Conception Vessel. This is called Small Circulation (Xiao Zhou Tian, 小周天). After mastering Small Circulation, you then learn "Grand Circulation" (Da Zhou Tian, 大周天) in which the mind guides the Qi through all of the twelve channels. This method has been practiced by Taijiquan devotees since the thirteenth century. Chapter 3 will explain Nei Dan practice in detail.

The third common way of increasing Qi circulation is through acupuncture. In acupuncture, a needle pierces the skin and musculature and directly stimulate a Qi channel. When the channel is stimulated, Qi builds up and circulates in that channel.

The fourth way is massage, which has also been used in Western medicine. Massage stimulates the muscles, building up local Qi, which circulates more freely because the muscles are relaxed.

The last common way is through friction, in which a particular area of the body is rubbed hard enough to generate heat and stimulate the skin.

There are a few other ways to build up local Qi, including slapping the skin and acupressure, which is classified somewhere between massage and acupuncture. Of the five most common methods mentioned above, Wai Dan and Nei Dan are the only two that can be applied to martial purposes. The others are for improving health, and will be explained in chapter 4.

1-4. Popular Martial Styles of Qigong Training

There are two categories of Qigong training: martial arts Qigong and Qigong for health, longevity, and spiritual attainment. Within each category there are many styles. The most popular non-martial Qigong methods are the Yi Jin Jing (易筋經) attributed to Da Mo (達磨) and Ba Duan Jin (Eight Pieces of Brocade, 八段錦). These are discussed in chapter 2.

The most popular martial arts used for Qigong are Taiji (太極), Xingyi (形意), Liu He Ba Fa (六合八法), and Bagua (八卦). Here we will give only a brief review of the history and theory; you should refer to a book or instructor of each style for deeper study. If you would like to know about Taiji, Xingyi, and Baguazhang, please refer to the books: The *Essence of Tai Chi Chi Kung—Hsing Yi Chuan* and *Baguazhang*, available from YMAA Publication Center.

Taijiquan

Taiji means "Grand Ultimate," and refers to the Yin—Yang concept in Chinese philosophy. Quan means "fist," "boxing," or "style." This boxing style is noted for its slow, relaxed movements. The forms are martial movements, but are performed very slowly, so they appear more like dance than like a martial art. Taiji is also know as Shi San Shi (十三勢) or Thirteen Postures, Mian Quan (綿拳) or Soft Sequence, and Changquan (長拳) or Long Sequence. "Thirteen Postures" refers to the thirteen principle techniques in Taijiquan that correspond to the eight trigrams combined with the five phases. These techniques are: Wardoff, Rollback, Press (or Squeeze), Push, Pluck, Rend, Elbow, and Bump for the eight trigrams, and Advance, Retreat, Dodge and Beware of the Left, Dodge and Beware of the Right, and Hold the Center for the five phases. "Soft Sequence" refers to the relaxed and gentle way in which the movements are performed. "Long Sequence" refers to the fact that the Taiji barehand sequence takes much longer to perform and contains a greater number of techniques than most other martial styles.

While there is little documentary evidence concerning the origins of Taijiquan, Zhang, San-Feng (張三豐) is generally credited with creating it at Wudang Mountain (武當山) during the Song dynasty (960-1280 A.D., 宋朝), basing it on the fighting techniques of the snake and crane combined with internal power. Until the mid-nineteenth century, Taijiquan was a closely guarded secret of the Chen family (陳家). At that time Yang, Lu-Shan (1780-1873 A.D.)(楊露禪) learned Taiji from Chen, Chang-Xing (陳長興), the grandmaster of that time. Yang went to Beijing and became famous as a martial artist, and passed the system on to his sons, who in turn passed it on to the public. Yang, Lu-Shan's second son, Yang, Ban-Hou (1837-1890 A.D.)(楊班侯) taught the style to a number of people, including Wu, Quan-You (吳全佑), whose son Wu, Jian-Quan (吳鑑泉) (Figure 1-4) modified the style and founded the Wu Style of Taijiquan (吳氏太極拳), which is especially popular in Hong Kong, Singapore, and Malaysia. A grandson of Yang, Lu-Shan, Yang, Cheng-Fu (1883-1935 A.D.) (楊澄甫) (Figure 1-5) formed the distinctive characteristics of what is now known as Yang Style Taijiquan (楊氏太極拳).

Concerning Qigong, Taiji has two aspects. One is moving meditation which consists of seventy-two to one hundred and twenty-eight martial forms (depending on the style and manner of counting) which are practiced in slow motion. During practice, the body is relaxed and the Qi generated at the Dan Tian is continuously guided by the will to circulate throughout the whole body. The second aspect is still meditation. Taiji meditation is a form of Daoist meditation, which will be explained in detail in chapter 3. Today the best known Taiji

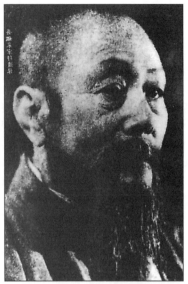

Figure 1-4. Wu, Jian-Quan

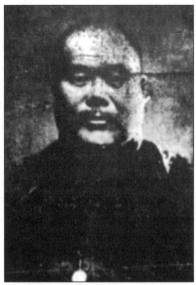

Figure 1-5. Yang, Chen-Fu

styles are Chen, Yang, and Wu. Each of these styles has subdivisions which emphasize different postures and applications.

Taijiquan also includes training with the sword, saber, spear, and staff to extend the Qi.

Baguazhang

Baguazhang (The Eight Trigrams Palm, 八卦掌), also known as Baguaquan (The Eight Trigrams Fist, 八卦拳), has a short history. It was created in Beijing by Dong, Hai-Chuan (董海川)(Figures 1-6 and 1-7), a native of Wen An district of Hebei province (河北文安), sometime between 1866 and 1880 A.D. According to several historical records, Dong learned his martial arts on Jiu Hua Mountain (九華山) from Bi, Cheng-Xia (畢澄霞). The style is a combination of the best features of the Shaolin (Buddhist) and Wudang (Daoist) martial arts. Baguazhang emphasizes the application of palm techniques and circular movements. It lays stress on the stability and consolidation of the stances and the flexibility of the waist, which is complimented by the swiftness of the arms and palms. When practicing, the devotee's mind controls the waist, and the waist controls the movement of the body in coordination with circular walking around an imagined center point. The movements of the three levels (low, center, and high) increase the practitioner's coordination, strength, and vigor.

The system includes two sets of palm techniques, Yin and Yang. The highest level of Baguazhang practice is called the Dragon Form. In this form the student moves not only in a circle around an imaginary center, but also rotates, twisting and turning, wheeling and moving vertically in combinations. The circular

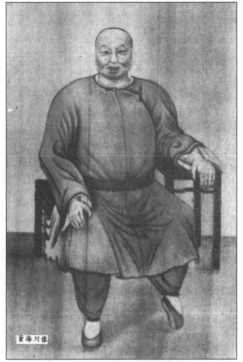

Figure 1-6. Dong, Hai-Chuan

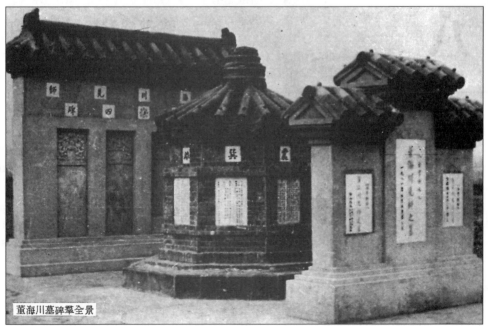

Figure 1-7. Tomb of Dong, Hai-Chuan in Beijing (rebuilt in 1981)

movements of Baguazhang are different from the straight line attack of Xingyiquan, but its fast motion and internal power training are the same, although both are different from Taijiquan and Liu He Ba Fa. If you are interested in studying more about Baguazhang, please refer to the book *Baguazhang—Emei Baguazhang*, available from YMAA Publication Center.

Xingyiquan

Xingyiquan (形意拳) (also spelled as Hsing Yi Chuan) consists of a set of fast punching movements. There are five basic punches based on the five basic motions: splitting (Pi, 劈), drilling (Zuan, 鑽), expanding (Beng, 弸), exploding (Pao, 砲), crossing (Heng, 橫). They are performed with the muscles first relaxed and then tensed, and the practitioner usually steps in a straight line while striking. In Chinese, Xing (形) means "shape" and Yi (意) means "mind," so Xingyi means "using the mind to determine the form." Marshal Yue Fei (岳飛) (1103-1141 A.D.) is popularly credited with creating Xingyiquan, although there is no documentary evidence to support the claim. It was not until the end of the Ming dynasty (1644 A.D., 明朝) that the documented history of Xingyiquan began. A martial artist named Ji, Long-Feng (姬隆豐) of Shanxi province (山西省) claimed to have obtained a book, *Quan Jing* (拳經) or *Fist Fighting Classic,* written by Yue Fei when he visited a hermit on Zhong Nan Mountain (終南山). The book describes martial techniques imitating the Dragon (龍), Tiger (虎), Monkey (猴), Horse (馬), Water Lizard (鼉), Chicken (雞), Harrier (鷂), Swallow (燕), Snake (蛇), Chinese Ostrich (鴕), Eagle and Bear (鷹，熊). After studying this book, Ji used his knowledge to develop the art and make a more complete style. In the three hundred years since then, other styles of Xingyiquan have been developed and practiced. Xingyiquan masters were frequently employed as caravan guards beginning in the 19th century.

Today there are at least ten sequences of Xingyiquan popularly practiced: Wu Xing Quan (五形拳), Shi Da Xing (十大形), Shi Er Xing (十二形), Ba Shi (八式), Za Shi Chui (雜式捶), Shi Er Heng Chui (十二橫捶), Chu Ru Dong (出入洞), An Shen Pao (安身炮), Jiao Shan Pao (絞山炮), and Wu Hua Pao (五花炮).

Xingyiquan is practiced at a fast speed, although with the muscles first relaxed and then tensed, and power is developed and concentrated in the Dan Tian (丹田). If you are interested in studying more about Xingyiquan, please refer to the book *Hsing Yi Chuan*, available from YMAA Publication Center.

Liu He Ba Fa

According to tradition, Liu He Ba Fa (六合八法) was created during the Song dynasty (960-1280 A.D., 宋朝) by Chen Bo (陳博), a hermit living on Hua Shan (Mount Hua, 華山). It combines the strategy and techniques of Taijiquan,

Xingyiquan, and Baguazhang. The training contains the soft within the hard and the hard within the soft. Its strategy employs straight line forward and backward movements as well as circular movements. It utilizes all three fighting ranges (short, middle, and long), but does not emphasize high kicking techniques. It is normally taught to those who have already learned the three previous styles, because they are more likely to understand the essence of the three and mix and apply the techniques skillfully and effectively. Liu He Ba Fa uses Liu He (The Six Combinations, 六合) as its theory and Ba Fa (The Eight Methods, 八法) as its practice. The Six Combinations are:

1. The body combines and coordinates with the mind.
2. The mind combines and coordinates with the idea.
3. The idea combines and coordinates with the Qi (inner energy, 氣)
4. The Qi (inner energy, 氣) combines and coordinates with the spirit (Shen, 神).
5. The spirit combines and coordinates with the movements.
6. The movements combine and coordinate with the universe.

These Six Combinations are achieved by means of The Eight Methods:

1. Qi (Breath, 氣): Controlling the breath through concentration.
2. Gu (Bone, 骨): Mustering force within the bones.
3. Xing (Shape, 形): Imitating the various forms and postures.
4. Sui (Following, 隨): Fluidly combining with the opponent's moves.
5. Ti (Lift, 提): Feeling that one is suspended by the top of the head.
6. Huan (Return, 還): Balancing motion and posture.
7. Le (Reserve, 勒): Maintaining peace and calmness of mind.
8. Fu (Conceal, 伏): Refraining from exposing one's intentions prematurely.

References

1. 莊子曰：〝真人之息以踵，眾人之息以喉。〞

2. Dr. Yang, Jwing-Ming. 1997. *The Root of Chinese Qigong, 2nd Edition.* YMAA Publication Center, Boston.

3. Robert O. Becker, M.D. and Gary Selden. 1985. *The Body Electric.* Quill, William Morrow, New York.

Chapter 2
Wai Dan Qigong
(External Elixir)
外丹氣功

2-1. Introduction

Wai Dan (pronounced "Why Dan," 外丹) is the practice of increasing Qi circulation by stimulating one area of the body until a large energy potential builds up and flows through the Qi channel system. In Chinese, the term Wai Dan also signifies the alchemical elixir of life (also called Jin Dan, 金丹), and it is probable that our use of the term derives from the alchemical usage. Most Chinese alchemical texts are products of the Daoists, who were a significant force in the development of Qigong, so it seems appropriate to call these Qigong training techniques that promote health, strength, and longevity by the Daoist name.

In this chapter, the principles of Wai Dan Qigong (外丹氣功) practice will be explained first. Then the most famous Shaolin Wai Dan training method, Da Mo's Yi Jin Jing (易筋經) will be introduced. Next, a number of other sets of Wai Dan training will be demonstrated, including the standing set of the well known Eight Pieces of Brocade (Ba Duan Jin, 八段錦). You should try all the exercises presented, then adopt a training schedule suited to your own needs. For example, you can pick one set and practice it every day for several months or even years, or do a different set every day. Your needs will change as you develop, so maintain a flexible attitude toward the training.

2-2. Principles of Wai Dan Qigong

There are two types of Wai Dan exercise, moving and still. In moving Wai Dan, a specific muscle or part of the body is repeatedly tensed and relaxed as you concentrate on that muscle. Use as little tension as possible because great tension will constrict the Qi channels and prevent the flow of energy. Some practitioners do not tense their muscles at all, but merely imagine tensing them. Others tense them just enough to aid concentration. When you exercise a part of the body in this way for several minutes, the Qi accumulates in that area, which usually results in a local feeling of warmth. Both energy and blood are collected in this high potential area. When the muscles relax, the highly charged Qi and blood will spread to nearby areas with a lower energy state and so increase the Qi circulation.

According to acupuncture theory, the Qi channels are connected to the internal organs. If Qi is circulating smoothly, then the organs will function normally. If an organ is not functioning normally, then increasing the Qi flow in the corresponding channel will help to restore its normal function.

In moving Wai Dan exercises, the mind concentrates on the breath and at the same time imagines guiding energy to a specific area. As was mentioned earlier, the Qi channel system and the brain are closely related, so that when you concentrate, you can control the circulation of Qi more efficiently. This in turn results in the muscles being able to exert maximum power. This is what is known as Wai Dan internal power. For example, in order to guide the Qi you have generated to the center of your palm, imagine an obstacle in front of your palm and try to push it away without tensing any muscles. The better you imagine, the stronger the Qi flow will be. Frequently, when an object seems too heavy to move, and you have tried in vain to push it, if you relax, calm down, and imagine pushing the object, you will find the object will now move. Therefore, in practicing the moving Wai Dan exercises, you should be calm, relaxed and natural. The muscles should never be strongly tensed, because this tension will narrow the Qi channels. Concentrate on breathing with the Dan Tian (Elixir Field, 丹田) and on guiding the Qi.

There is a disadvantage to Wai Dan moving exercises. Because of the repeated tensing and relaxing of the muscles during training, the muscle itself will be built up, as in weight lifting, and can become overdeveloped. This over development will slow you down, and at the same time will constrict the channels. When these overdeveloped muscles are not regularly exercised, they accumulate fat, which will further narrow the channels, and the Qi and blood will become stagnant. Common symptoms of this phenomenon are high blood pressure, local nerve pain, and poor muscle control. In the Chinese martial arts this is called San Gong (散功) or Energy Dispersion. As long as you avoid overdeveloping your muscles, San Gong will not happen.

In still Wai Dan, specific muscle groups are also stressed, but they are not tensed. For example, in one type of still Wai Dan practice you extend both arms level in front of your body and hold the posture. After several minutes the nerves in the arms and shoulder areas become excited, and reach a higher energy state. When you drop your arms and relax, the generated Qi will circulate to areas of lower potential, much like an electric battery circulates electricity when a circuit is made. In still Wai Dan, there is no danger of over development because the muscle is not being exercised as it is in moving Wai Dan, so consequently there is no risk of San Gong. Although the muscle is not built up in still Wai Dan training, its endurance is increased.

If you practice Wai Dan and also have training in Nei Dan (internal elixir, 內丹), you can accumulate Qi in the Dan Tian with breathing and concentration, and guide this energy to the area being stressed to enhance the Qi circulation. In this case the method is a mixture of Wai Dan and Nei Dan. This kind of training is commonly used in the practice of Taijiquan.

2-3. Da Mo's Yi Jin Jing Exercises

Da Mo (Figure 2-l), whose last name was Chadili (刹帝利), and who was also known as Bodhidarma, was a prince of a small tribe in southern India. From the fragments of historical records that exist it is believed he was born about 483 A.D. At that time India was considered a spiritual center by the Chinese, since it was the source of Buddhism, which was becoming very influential in China. Many of the Chinese emperors either sent priests to India to study Buddhism and bring back scriptures, or else they invited Indian priests to come to China to preach. Da Mo was an invited priest.

He is considered by many to have been a bodhisattva, or an enlightened being who had renounced nir-

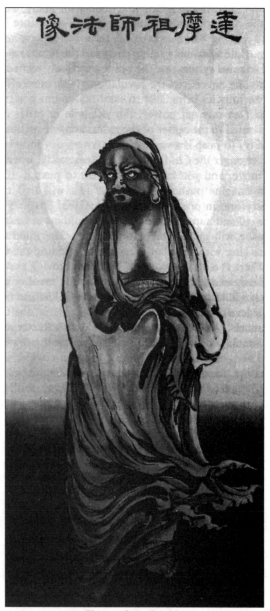

Figure 2-1. Da Mo

vana in order to save others. Briefly, Buddhism is a major religion based on the belief that Gautama, the Buddha, achieved nirvana, or perfect bliss and freedom from the cycle of birth and death, and taught how to achieve this state. Buddhists are divided into three principal groups practicing different versions of the Buddha's teaching, which are called the "Three Conveyances or San Sheng (三乘). The first of these is Mahayana or Da Sheng (大乘), the Great

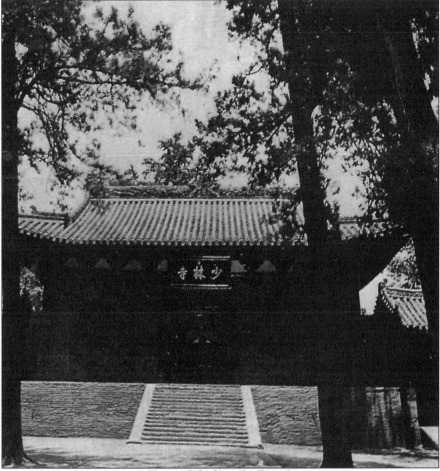

Figure 2-2. Shaolin Temple

Vehicle, which includes Tibetan Buddhism and Chan (禪) or Zen (忍) Buddhism, which is very well known to the West. The second is Praktika or Zhong Sheng (中乘), the Middle Way, which is the Buddhism of action, and is mostly practiced by wandering preachers. The third is Hinayana or Xiao Sheng (小乘), the Lesser Conveyance, which is generally practiced by ascetic monks and aims for the personal achievement of enlightenment.

Da Mo was of the Mahayana school and came to China in 526 or 527 A.D. during the reign of Emperor Liang Wu of the Liang dynasty (梁武帝). He went first to the Guang Xiao Temple in Canton (廣東光孝寺). The governor of Canton, Xiao Ang (蕭昂) recommended Da Mo to the emperor, who invited Da Mo to visit. The emperor, however, did not like Da Mo's Buddhist theory, and so Da Mo traveled to the Shaolin Temple (少林寺)(Figure 2-2) in Henan province (河南省) where he spent the rest of his life.

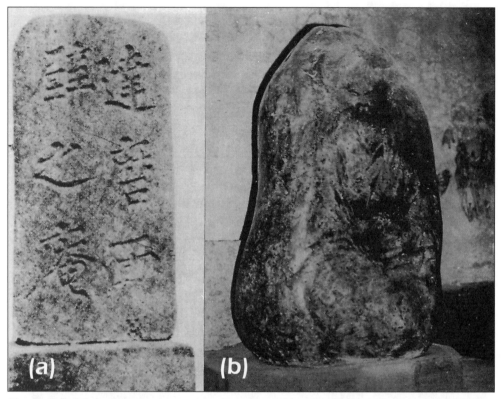

Figure 2-3. (a) A stone monument at the place where Da Mo faced the wall in meditation. (b) A rock with Da Mo's image found at the place where he meditated.

The Shaolin Temple was built around 400 A.D. on the Shao Shi (少室) peak of Song Mountain (嵩山) in Deng Feng Xian (登封縣), Henan province (河南省), by order of Emperor Wei (魏). It was built for a Buddhist named Batuo (跋陀法師) for the purpose of preaching and worship. In the beginning no martial arts training was done by the monks.

When Da Mo arrived at the temple, he saw that the monks were generally in poor physical condition because of their lack of exercise. He was so distressed by the situation that he retired to meditate on the problem, and stayed in retirement for nine years (Figure 2-3). During that time he wrote two books—the *Yi Jin Jing (Muscle/Tendon Changing Classic,* 易筋經) and *Xi Sui Jing (Marrow/Brain Washing Classic,* 洗髓經). After he came out of retirement, Da Mo continued to live in the Shaolin Temple until his death in 540 A.D. at the age of fifty-seven.

Lu You (陸游), a poet of the Southern Song dynasty (1127-1280 A.D., 南宋), wrote a poem describing Da Mo's personal philosophy:

宋陸游爲達磨詩

亦不覩惡而生嫌。亦不觀善而勤措。

亦不捨智而近愚。亦不拋迷而就悟。

達大道兮過量，通佛心兮出度，

不與凡聖同經，超然名之曰祖。

Feeling not disgusted by corruption and evil,

Nor eager grasping after desire and gain,

Sacrificing not wisdom for the company of fools,

Nor abandoning wonder to preserve the truth,

Reaching the great Dao without excessiveness,

Attaining the Buddha heart without vindictiveness,

Keeping not to the path of mere normal holiness,

Transcendent of its own creation.

For more than fourteen hundred years, the monks of the Shaolin Temple have trained using the Da Mo Wai Dan exercises. These exercises used to be secret, and only in the twentieth century have they become popularly known and used by the Chinese people. These exercises are easy and their benefits are experienced in a short time. The Shaolin monks practice these exercises not just to circulate Qi and improve their health, but also to build their internal power by concentrating Qi to affect the appropriate muscles. Because these exercises are moving Wai Dan, there is the risk of San Gong or Energy Dispersion, as mentioned earlier. To avoid San Gong, the monks also practice Nei Dan meditation to keep their Qi channels clear after they stop practicing the Da Mo exercises.

When practicing the Da Mo exercises, find a place with clean air, stand facing the east with your back relaxed and naturally straight, and your feet shoulder-width apart and parallel. Facing the east takes advantage of the earth's rotation and the energy flow from the sun. Keeping the legs apart will relax the legs and thighs during practice. Keep your mouth closed and touch your palate with the tip of the tongue without strain. In Chinese meditation this touch is called Da Qiao (搭橋) or Building the Bridge because it connects the Yin and Yang circulation (a detailed explanation of this will follow in chapter 3). Saliva will accumulate in your mouth, swallow it to keep your throat from getting dry.

The key to successful practice of this exercise is concentrating on the area being exercised, and concentrating on your breath. Without this concentration, the original goal of Qi circulation will be lost and the exercise will be in vain.

There are several circumstances when practice should be avoided. Do not practice when you are very hungry or too full. If you are very hungry it interferes with proper concentration. If you have eaten, wait at least thirty minutes, and preferably one hour before practicing so that the Qi is not so concentrated in the digestive system. Avoid practicing one day before or after having sex. Do not practice when you are so tired that your attention wanders uncontrollably. Do not practice after drinking alcohol. And finally, do not practice when you are very worried, for it will be too difficult to concentrate.

The forms should be done continuously, one after the other, in order to conserve the energy you build up. For example, the first form will build up the energy at the wrist. The second form will transfer the energy already built up at the wrist to the fingers and palms while continuing to build up energy. The third form will transfer the energy from the palms and wrists to the arms, and so forth.

Repeat each form fifty times. A repetition consists of inhaling while relaxing the muscle or limb and then exhaling while imagining that you are tightening the muscle and imagining energy flowing to that area. The muscles may be *slightly* tensed. The arms should not be fully extended in these forms. After fifty repetitions, begin the next form in the sequence without stopping.

Beginners may find it hard to complete more than five forms if they do fifty repetitions of each form. Do not be concerned. Five forms is a good number to practice because this means a practice session will take approximately fifteen to twenty minutes. Alternatively, you can practice all twelve forms and do fewer repetitions of each. For example, twenty repetitions of each form of the complete Da Mo set would take approximately twenty minutes. If you practice once or twice a day, you should be able to complete the entire form in six months. If you continue this training for three years, you can build a tremendous amount of power and energy. These exercises will increase the nerve and muscle efficiency so they can be used to their maximum in martial arts. If you are practicing for health purposes only, five forms daily is sufficient.

Da Mo Wai Dan 達磨外丹

Form 1 (Figure 2-4). Keep your hands beside your body with the palms open and facing down, fingertips pointing forward. Keep the elbows bent. Imagine pushing the palms down and lifting your fingers backward when exhaling, and relax them when inhaling. This form will build the Qi or energy at the wrist area, and your palms and wrists should feel warm after fifty repetitions.

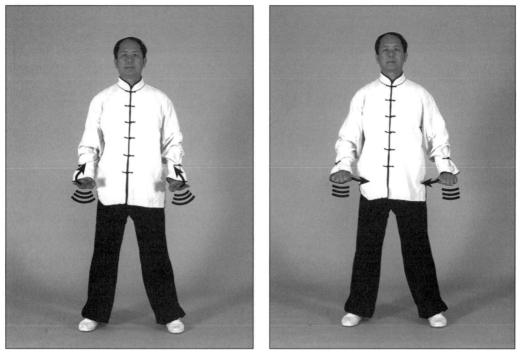

Figure 2-4   Figure 2-5

Form 2 (Figure 2-5). Without moving your arms, make fists with palms facing down and thumbs extended toward the body. Imagine tightening your fists and pushing the thumbs backwards when exhaling, and then relax when inhaling. Keep your wrists bent to retain the energy built up in the first form.

Form 3 (Figure 2-6). Again without moving your arms, turn the fists so that the palms face each other, and place the thumbs over the fingers, like a normal fist. Imagine tightening your fists when exhaling, and relax when inhaling. The muscles and nerves of the arms will be stimulated and energy will accumulate there.

Form 4 (Figure 2-7). Extend your arms straight forward at shoulder height, palms still facing each other. Making normal fists, imagine tightening when exhaling, and then relaxing when inhaling. This will build up energy in the shoulders and chest.

Form 5 (Figure 2-8). Lift your arms straight up, palms facing each other, keeping the fists. Imagine tightening the fists when exhaling and relaxing when inhaling. This builds energy in the shoulders, neck and sides.

Form 6 (Figure 2-9). Lower your arms so that the upper arms are parallel to the ground, the elbows are bent, and your fists are by your ears. The palms face forward. Imagine tightening the fists when exhaling, and relaxing when inhaling. This builds energy in the sides, chest, and upper arms.

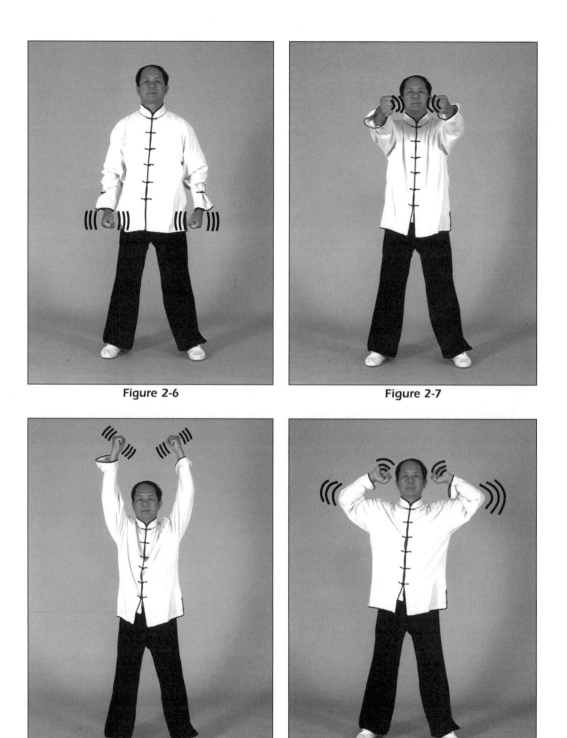

Figure 2-6

Figure 2-7

Figure 2-8

Figure 2-9

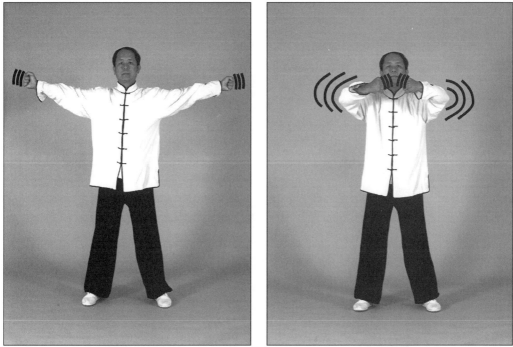

Figure 2-10   Figure 2-11

Form 7 (Figure 2-10). Extend the arms straight out to the sides with the palms facing forward. Imagine tightening your fists when exhaling and relaxing them when inhaling. This form will build energy in the shoulders, chest, and back.

Form 8 (Figure 2-11). Hold your arms in front of your body at shoulder height with the palms facing in, and your elbows slightly bent to create a rounded effect with the arms. Imagine tightening the fists and guiding the accumulated energy through the arms to the fists when exhaling; relax when inhaling.

Form 9 (Figure 2-12). Pull your fists toward your body, bending the elbows. Keep your fists just in front of your face, with the palms facing out. Imagine tightening your fists when exhaling, and then relax when inhaling. This form is similar to Form 6, but the fists are closer together and forward, so a different set of muscles is stressed. This form intensifies the flow of energy through the arms.

Form 10 (Figure 2-l3). Lift your forearms vertically. Your palms face forward and your upper arms are out to the sides and parallel with the floor. Imagine tightening your fists when exhaling, and then relax when inhaling. This form will circulate the energy built up in the shoulders.

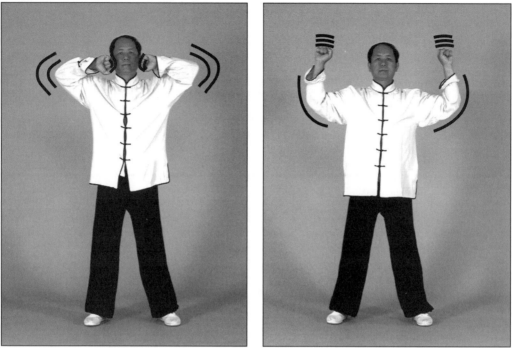

Figure 2-12	**Figure 2-13**

Form 11 (Figure 2-14). Keeping your elbows bent, lower your fists until they are in front of the navel, palms down. Imagine tightening your fists, and guide the energy to circulate in the arms when exhaling. Relax when inhaling. This is the first recovery form.

Form 12 (Figure 2-15). Hold your arms straight out in front of your body. Open your hands so that your palms face up. Imagine lifting up when exhaling, and then relax when inhaling. This is the second recovery form.

After practicing, stand for a few minutes with your arms hanging loosely at your sides. You can also lie down and relax completely. Breathe regularly, relax, and feel the energy redistribute itself.

2-4. Other Popular Wai Dan Exercises

There are many other sets of Wai Dan exercises derived from Da Mo's sequence. In this section the most common Wai Dan sets will be introduced. These are the Open Palm Sequence, which moves power to the fingertips; Moving Forms for coordinating breathing with movement of the arms, legs, and trunk; and Eight Pieces of Brocade, a set of simple exercises well known throughout China. In addition, a set of Still Forms that can be used to develop stamina and flexibility are included.

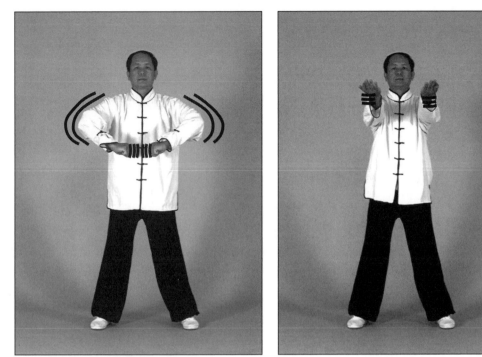

Figure 2-14   Figure 2-15

Open Palm Sequence

The open palm forms train you to extend energy to the palms and fingertips. In this set, keep your hands open. The thumbs and little fingers are pulled back and tightened slightly so that energy is directed to the centers of the palms. To understand how to do this, imagine holding a basketball or large balloon in both hands without the thumbs or little fingers touching it.

This set of exercises has the same purpose as the Da Mo Wai Dan set, so the same rules and principles should be followed. However, instead of tensing your fists, the palms are tensed and the energy is continuously guided to the fingertips.

Form 1 (Figure 2-16). Your palms face the floor while your fingers point out to the sides. Imagine pushing down when exhaling, then relax when inhaling.

Form 2 (Figure 2-17). Your palms face your legs, fingers pointing down. Imagine pushing in towards your body when exhaling, then relax when inhaling.

Form 3 (Figure 2-18). Extend your arms out to the sides, palms facing up. Imagine pushing up when exhaling, then relax when inhaling.

Form 4 (Figure 2-19). Bend your arms and place your hands in front of your chest, palms facing each other, fingers pointing up. Imagine pushing your hands toward each other when exhaling, then relax when inhaling.

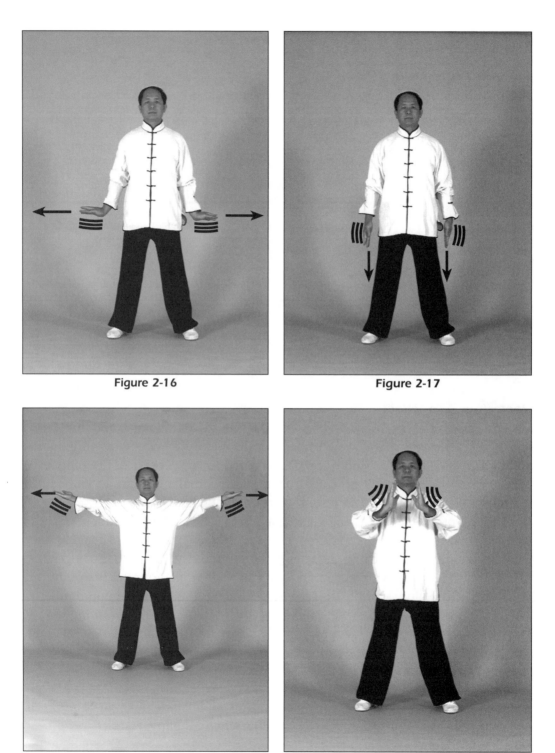

Figure 2-16

Figure 2-17

Figure 2-18

Figure 2-19

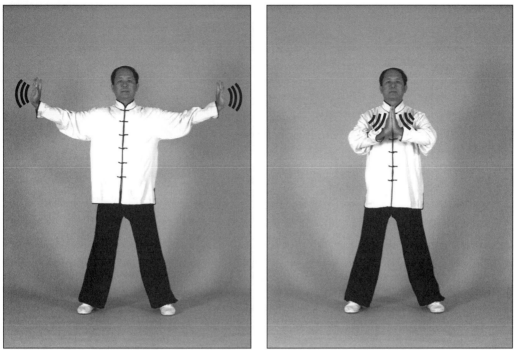

Figure 2-20   Figure 2-21

Form 5 (Figure 2-20). Extend your arms out to the sides, palms facing out, fingers pointing up. Imagine pushing out when exhaling, then relax when inhaling.

Form 6 (Figure 2-21). Bend your arms and place your hands in front of your chest again, this time with the palms touching. Imagine pushing in when exhaling, then relax when inhaling.

Form 7 (Figure 2-22). Extend your arms straight out in front of your body at shoulder height, palms facing forward, fingers pointing up. Imagine pushing forward when exhaling, then relax when inhaling.

Form 8 (Figure 2-23). Lift your arms straight up, palms facing up, fingers pointing toward each other. Imagine pushing up when exhaling, then relax when inhaling.

Form 9 (Figure 2-24). Lower your hands in front of your chest, elbows bent, palms facing up, fingers pointing toward each other. Imagine lifting up when exhaling, then relax when inhaling.

Form 10 (Figure 2-25). Extend your arms straight out in front of your body, palms facing up, fingers pointing forward. Imagine pushing up when exhaling, then relax when inhaling.

Form 11 (Figure 2-26). Bring your hands in front of your chest, palms facing down, fingers lined up and almost touching. Imagine pushing down when exhaling, then relax when inhaling.

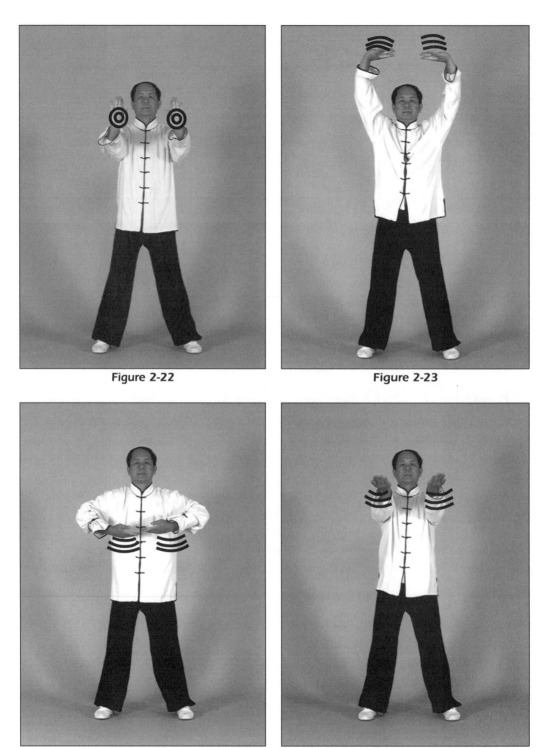

Figure 2-22

Figure 2-23

Figure 2-24

Figure 2-25

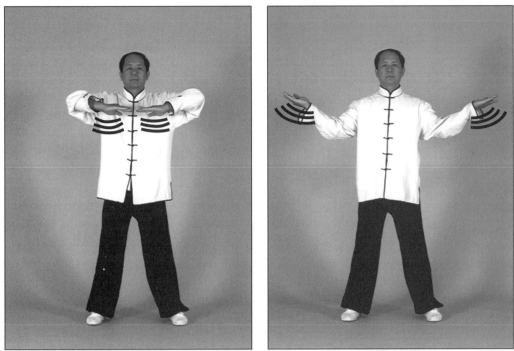

Figure 2-26   Figure 2-27

Form 12 (Figure 2-27). Extend your arms out to the sides with the elbows bent, palms facing up and slightly inward. Imagine lifting upward and inward when exhaling, and then relax when inhaling.

Just as with the Da Mo Wai Dan, after practicing stand for a few minutes with your arms hanging loosely at your sides. You can also lie down and relax completely. Breathe regularly, relax, and feel the energy redistribute itself.

Moving Forms

The Moving Forms train large muscle coordination, develop the large muscles, and loosen the joints, particularly the back. These forms are a new development in Qigong and were created because practitioners felt that the Yi Jin Jing forms emphasized the arms to the exclusion of the rest of the body. When practicing, repeat each form five to ten times.

Form 1 (Figures 2-28 and 2-29). Stand erect with your arms at your sides and your feet shoulder width apart. Bend forward and touch your fingertips to the floor. Keep your knees straight, if possible, then return to a standing posture. Exhale when bending forward, and inhale while straightening up.

Form 2 (Figures 2-30 and 2-31). Stand up and hold your palms in front of your chest and facing each other. While exhaling, bring your hands together until they almost touch. When you inhale let the hands separate. As you bring your hands together, imagine energy flowing to the palms, completing a circuit.

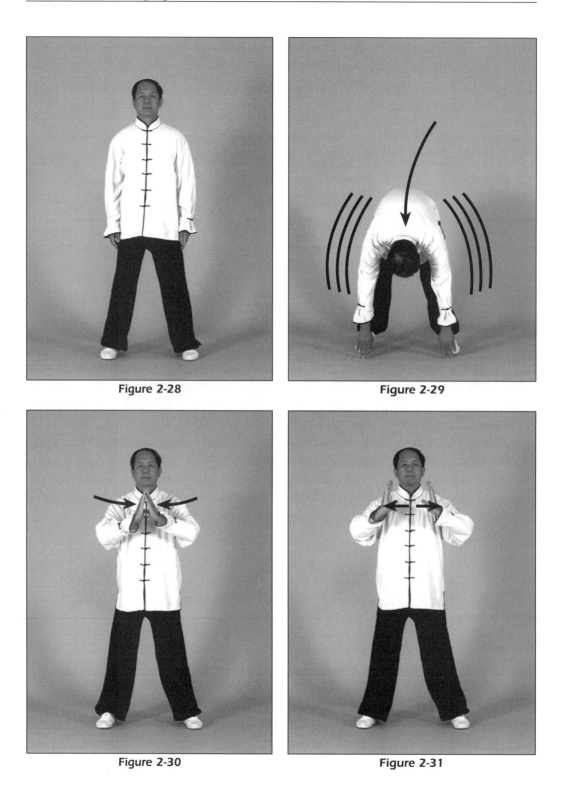

Figure 2-28

Figure 2-29

Figure 2-30

Figure 2-31

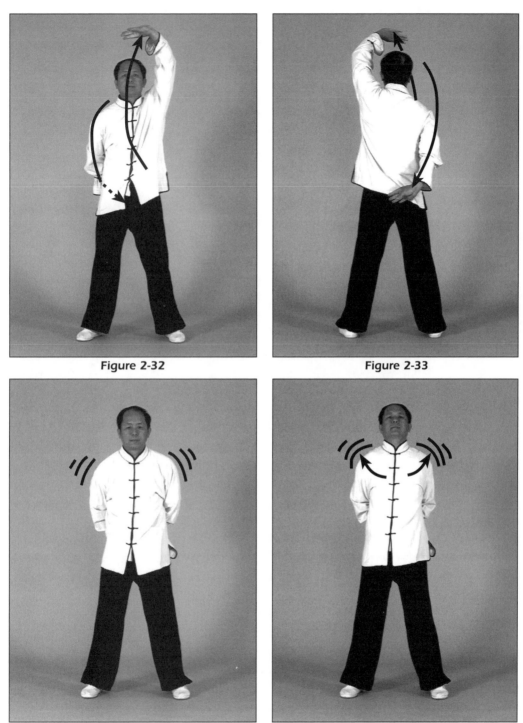

Figure 2-32

Figure 2-33

Figure 2-34

Figure 2-35

Form 3 (Figures 2-32 and 2-33). Exhale and push one palm straight up over your head while pushing down behind your back with the other palm. Relax and

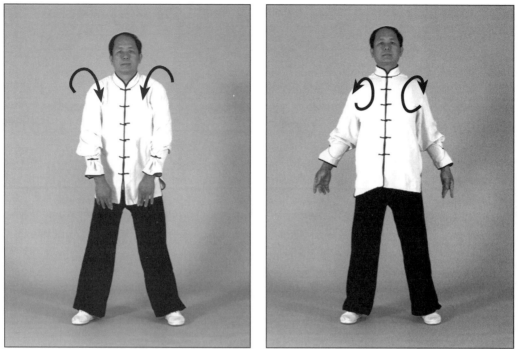

Figure 2-36   Figure 2-37

inhale while reversing the position of your hands.

Form 4 (Figures 2-34 and 2-35). Clasp your hands behind your back. Expand your chest when inhaling and relax while exhaling.

Form 5 (Figures 2-36 and 2-37). Stand with your arms hanging at your sides. Rotate your shoulders together ten times in one direction, then ten times in the other. Coordinate the movement with your breathing. It doesn't matter whether you inhale as the shoulders are moving forward or backward, as long as you are consistent.

Form 6 (Figure 2-38). Reach behind your back with the left hand and reach over your shoulder with the right hand and clasp hands. Expand your chest while inhaling, and relax when exhaling. Do this ten times, then reverse your arms and do ten more times.

Form 7 (Figures 2-39 to 2-41). Clasp your hands behind your back while standing, and then turn your torso from side to side while in a half squat. Exhale while turning to each side and inhale as you turn to the center.

Form 8 (Figures 2-42 and 2-43). Stand in a half squat with your arms out to the sides and your elbows slightly bent. While inhaling, turn your palms up and lift upward, and while exhaling turn your palms over and push down.

Form 9 (Figures 2-44 and 2-45). Bend forward. When inhaling, touch the backs of your hands to the floor, and when exhaling remain bent over and press down on the back of your neck with your palms. You may bend your knees slightly.

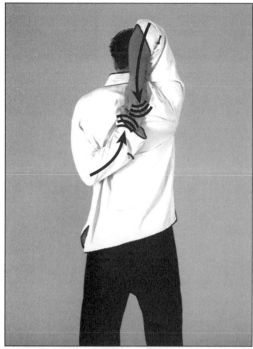

Figure 2-38

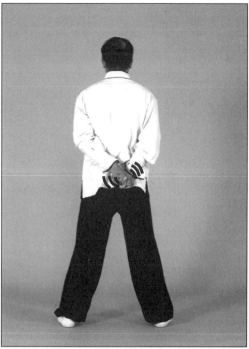

Figure 2-39

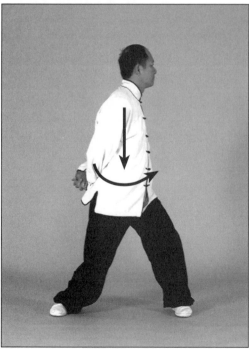

Figure 2-40

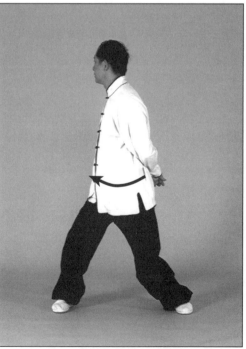

Figure 2-41

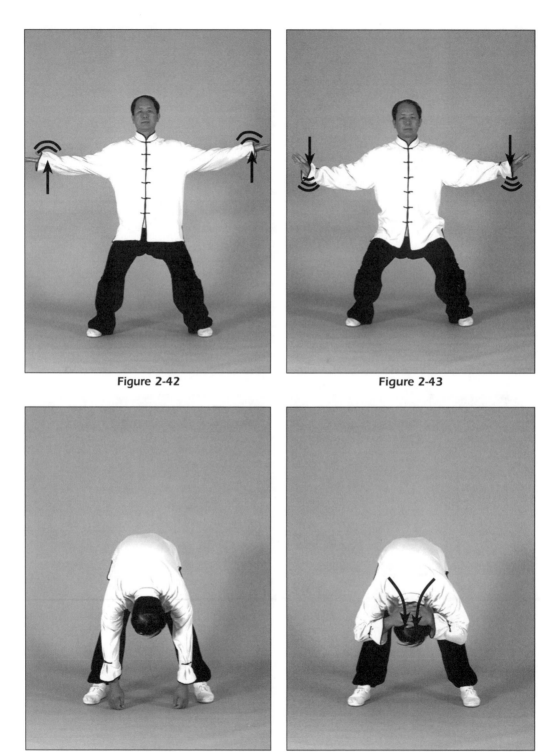

Figure 2-42

Figure 2-43

Figure 2-44

Figure 2-45

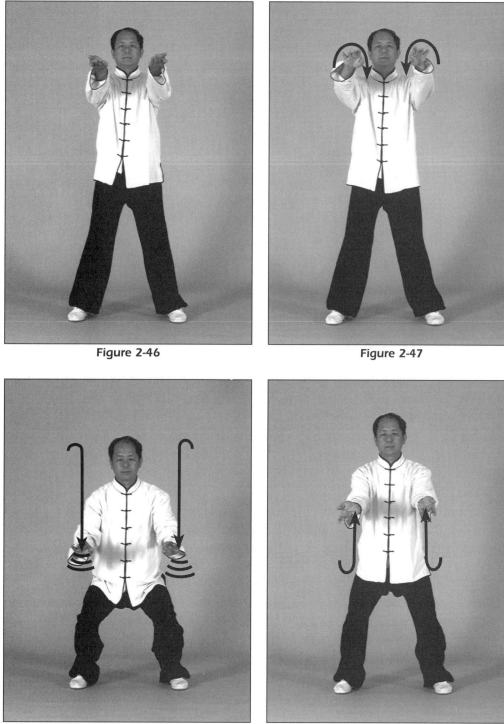

Figure 2-46

Figure 2-47

Figure 2-48

Figure 2-49

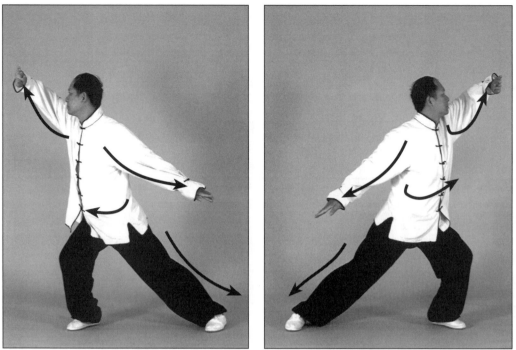

Figure 2-50   Figure 2-51

Form 10 (Figures 2-46 to 2-49). Stand with your arms extended straight in front of you, palms up. When exhaling, turn the palms down and lower your body by bending your knees, and when inhaling turn the palms up and stand back up.

Form 11 (Figures 2-50 and 2-51). Stand with your feet as far apart as is comfortable. Shift most of your weight to your right foot, and at the same time turn to the right, raising your right arm diagonally upward, palm facing out and up. Point the fingers of your left hand in the opposite direction. Think of the two arms as one unit forming a straight line. Then reverse positions, shifting most of your weight to your left foot, and at the same time turning to the left, raising your left arm diagonally upward, palm facing out and up. Point the fingers of your right hand in the opposite direction. Exhale while turning, and inhale while changing sides.

Form 12 (Figures 2-52 and 2-53). Stand with your feet as far apart as is comfortable. Shift most of your weight to your left foot, and at the same time turn to the left, bending the body sideways with the right arm in front of your head, and the left arm behind your back. The upper palm faces out while the lower palm faces downward. Twist to the left as far as possible with the feeling of spiraling, or pushing, through both hands. Then reverse the posture, shifting most

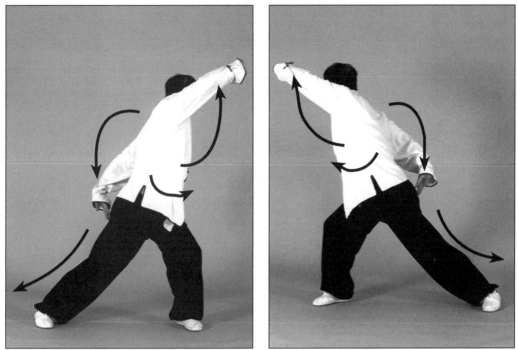

| Figure 2-52 | Figure 2-53 |

of your weight to your right foot and at the same time turning to the right, reversing the arms. Exhale while stretching, and inhale while changing sides.

Standing Eight Pieces of Brocade

Marshal Yue Fei (岳飛) is credited with creating the Eight Pieces of Brocade (Ba Duan Jin, 八段錦) in the twelfth century, during the Song dynasty (960-1280 A.D., 宋朝), in order to improve the health of his soldiers. The original set consisted of twelve forms, but this has been shortened to eight. This set is widely practiced all over China, and several distinct styles have developed, all of them effective. The name comes from brocade, which is a cloth, usually of silk, woven into complex and colorful patterns. Brocade is very highly prized, just as the good health produced by these simple exercises is prized.

Because this set was created nearly one thousand years ago, many versions exist. Only one of these versions is presented in this book. If you have learned or seen a different version, do not be concerned. The principles and the goals of the practice remain the same. If you are interested in knowing more about the theory and practice of the Eight Pieces of Brocade, please refer to the book *Eight Simple Qigong Exercises for Health*, available from YMAA Publication Center.

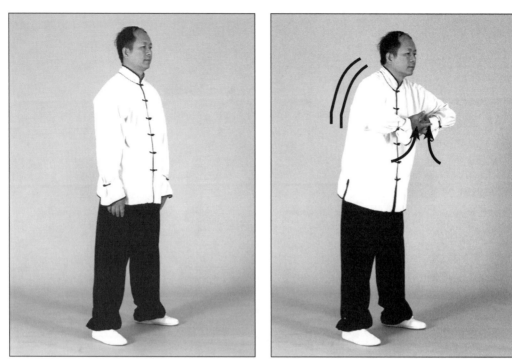

Figure 2-54   Figure 2-55

When performing the set, observe the following rules:

1. Relax before and after exercising, perhaps by taking a short walk.

2. Breathe naturally through your nose.

3. Keep your back vertical, except where leaning is part of the exercise.

4. Practice where ventilation is good and the air is fresh.

5. Perform the exercises slowly and stay relaxed.

6. For beginners, repeat each piece at least six times. Once your health and strength improves, continue to increase the number of repetitions until you can do each piece twenty-four times.

Piece 1 (Figures 2-54 to 2-58). Stand naturally, with your feet parallel and shoulder width apart, and your hands at your sides. Close your eyes, calm your mind, and breathe regularly. Open your eyes and look forward, and continue breathing naturally and smoothly. Condense your Shen (spirit) in your third eye (located in the center of your forehead), and sink your Qi to the Dan Tian. Then interlock your fingers and raise your hands above your head without bending your arms, and at the same time lift your heels. This is called Double Hands Hold up the Heavens (Shuang Shou Tuo Tian, 雙手托天). Drop your heels, and tilt your body to the left and then to the right, and then stand

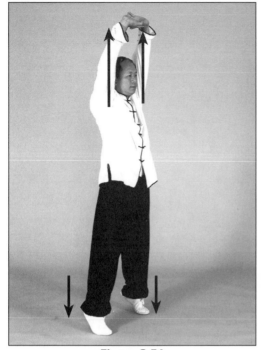

Figure 2-56

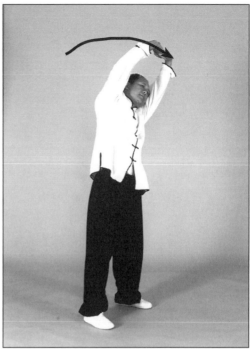

Figure 2-57

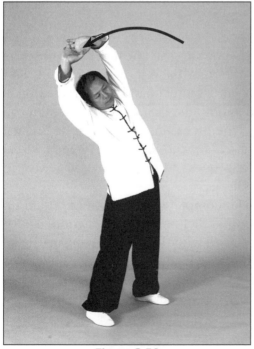

Figure 2-58

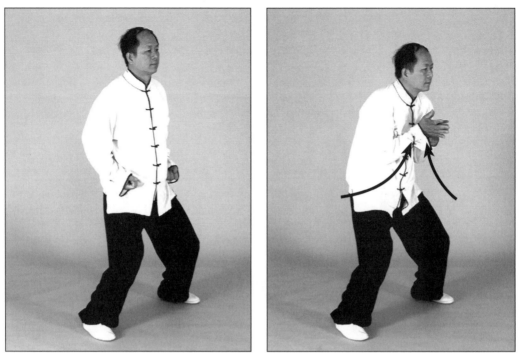

Figure 2-59   Figure 2-60

up straight again. Lower your hands in front of your body to complete the piece. Do twenty-four repetitions.

Piece 2 (Figures 2-59 to 2-63). Step to the right with your right leg, and squat down slightly. Relax your hands and lift them up to the chest area. Bring your palms together, then separate them with the right hand moving near the right nipple. Your left hand changes into the "sword secret" hand form and extends to the left as if you were pulling a bow to shoot a hawk. (To do the hand form, close all of your fingers into a fist except the index finger and middle finger). Stare at a distant point to your left. Then stand up and lower your hands, circle them up to the chest and repeat the same process to your right. Do twelve in either direction for a total of twenty-four pieces.

Piece 3 (Figures 2-64 to 2-67). After you complete the last piece, stand up and move your legs so that your feet are parallel and shoulder width apart. Then move both hands in front of your stomach with the palms facing up. Raise your left hand above your head and push upward, and at the same time lower your right hand to your right side, palm down, and press down slightly. Then change your hands and repeat the same process. You should feel that both

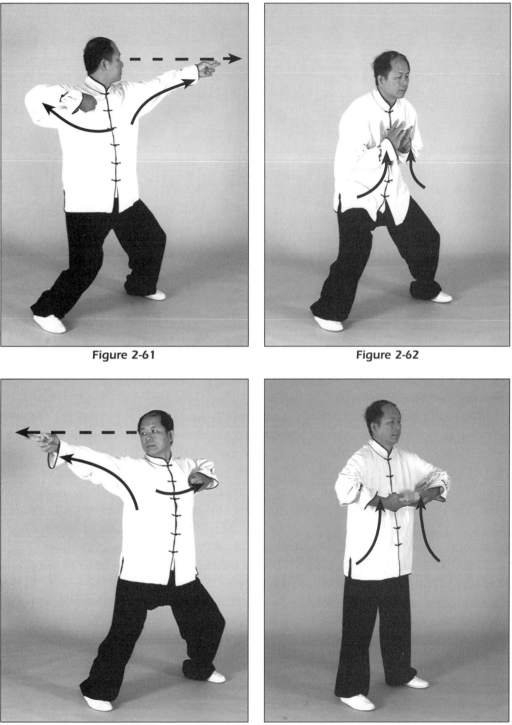

Figure 2-61

Figure 2-62

Figure 2-63

Figure 2-64

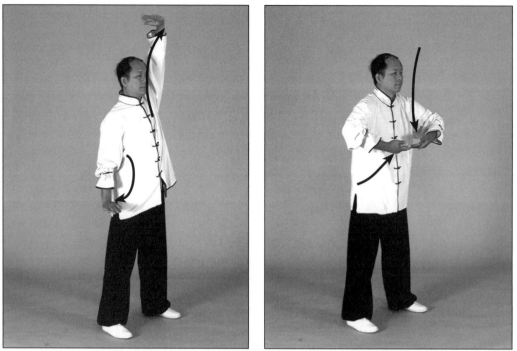

Figure 2-65   Figure 2-66

hands are pushing against resistance, but you must not tense your muscles. Do twenty-four repetitions.

Piece 4 (Figures 2-68 to 2-74). Stand easily and comfortably with both feet parallel as before, and your hands hanging down naturally at your sides. Lift your chest slightly from the inside so that your posture is straight, but be careful not to thrust your chest out. Turn your head to the left and look over your shoulder as you exhale, then turn your head to the front as you inhale. Turn your head to the right and look over your shoulder as you exhale, then again turn your head to the front as you inhale. Turn twelve times in each direction, for a total of twenty-four. Only turn your head. Your body does not move.

Next, place your hands on your lower back and turn your head twenty-four times as before. Finally, move both hands to your chest with the palms facing up, hold your elbows and shoulders slightly forward, and repeat the head turns another twenty-four times.

During all three parts, when you exhale and turn your head, use your mind to lead the Qi from the Dan Tian, approximately an inch and a half below your

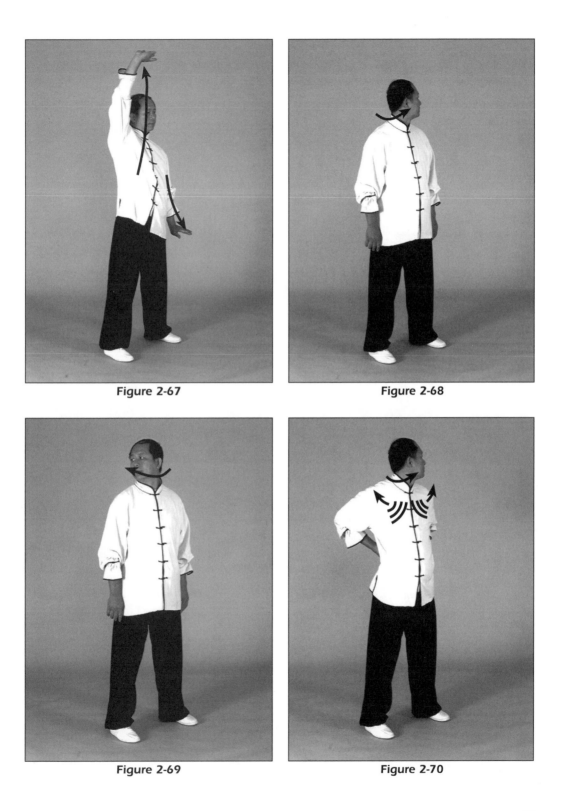

Figure 2-67

Figure 2-68

Figure 2-69

Figure 2-70

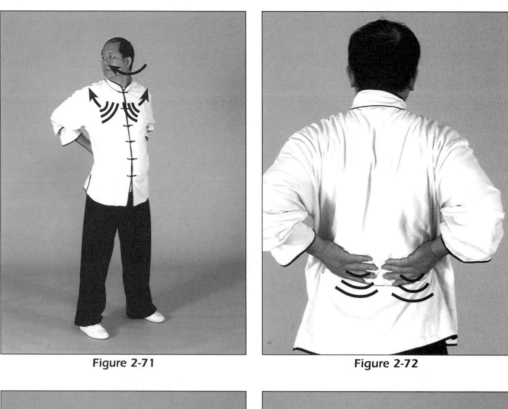

Figure 2-71

Figure 2-72

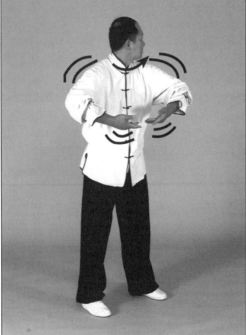

Figure 2-73

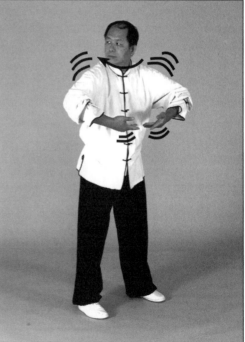

Figure 2-74

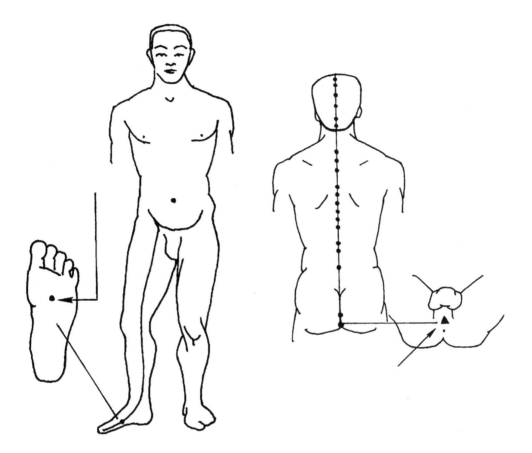

**Figure 2-75 Bubbling Well
Cavity (Yongquan)**

Figure 2-76 Huiyin Cavity

navel, to your Bubbling Well cavity (Yongquan) (Figure 2-75) and Huiyin cavity
(Figure 2-76). Then, as you turn your head to the front and inhale, lead the Qi
back to the Dan Tian.

Piece 5 (Figures 2-77 to 2-80). Take one step to the right with your right leg
and squat down. Place your hands on top of your knees, with the thumbs on the
outside of the thighs. Sink your Qi to the bottoms of your feet, and place your
mind on the two Bubbling Well cavities (one on each foot). Shift your weight to
your left leg and press down heavily with your hand, and line up (i.e. extend)
your head, spine, and right leg. Stay in this position for about three seconds,

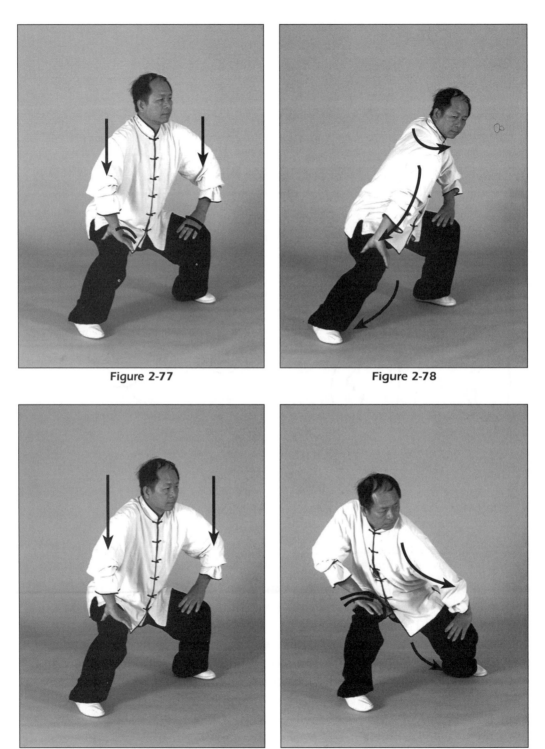

Figure 2-77

Figure 2-78

Figure 2-79

Figure 2-80

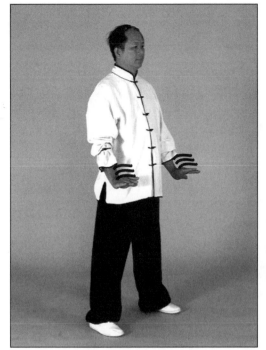

Figure 2-81

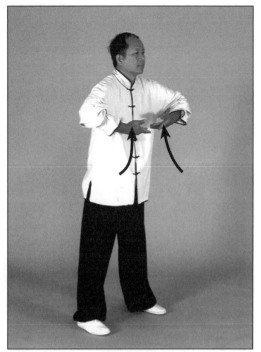

Figure 2-82

then return to the original position, and then repeat the same thing on the other side. Turn twelve times in each direction for a total of twenty-four repetitions.

Piece 6 (Figures 2-81 to 2-85). Move your left leg back so that your feet are shoulder width apart. Press both palms down beside your waist, then move your hands up in front of your chest and above your head with the palms facing up. The form looks as if you were holding or lifting something above your head. Stay there for three seconds, then bend forward, extend your arms, and hold your feet. Pull your hands up slightly so that you are putting a gentle stress on your whole body. While holding your feet, your

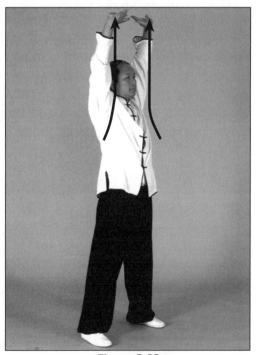

Figure 2-83

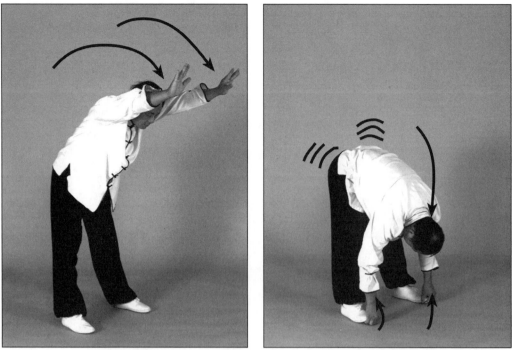

Figure 2-84   Figure 2-85

mind is on the Bubbling Well cavities. Stay there for three seconds. Repeat the entire process sixteen times.

Piece 7 (Figures 2-86 to 2-89). This piece is very similar to the second piece. Step out to your right and squat down, holding your body erect and your fists beside your waist. Tighten both fists, and extend one arm to the side in a twisting, punching motion (i.e. screw the fist). Your other hand stays beside your waist in a tight fist. The hand that is out can be either a fist or an open palm. After you finish the extending movement, loosen both hands and bring the extended hand back to your waist to the starting position. Then tighten both hands and repeat on the other side. When you make the punching motion, glare fiercely at an imaginary opponent. Remember to punch slowly. Do eight on either side, for a total of sixteen.

Piece 8 (Figures 2-90 to 2-96). There are three parts to this piece. First, let both hands drop down naturally beside your body. Stand still and keep your mind calm. Lift yourself up on your toes and stay as high as you can for three seconds. Then lower your feet to the floor. Repeat twenty-four times. Next, place your hands on your lower back, and again lift yourself up on your toes for three seconds, and then let yourself down. Also do this twenty-four times. Finally, hold your hands in front of your chest and again lift yourself twenty-four times. The different hand positions serve different Qi circulation functions.

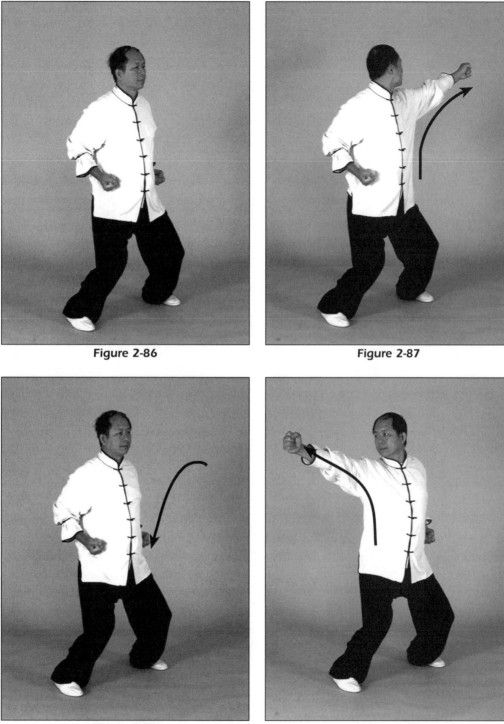

Figure 2-86

Figure 2-87

Figure 2-88

Figure 2-89

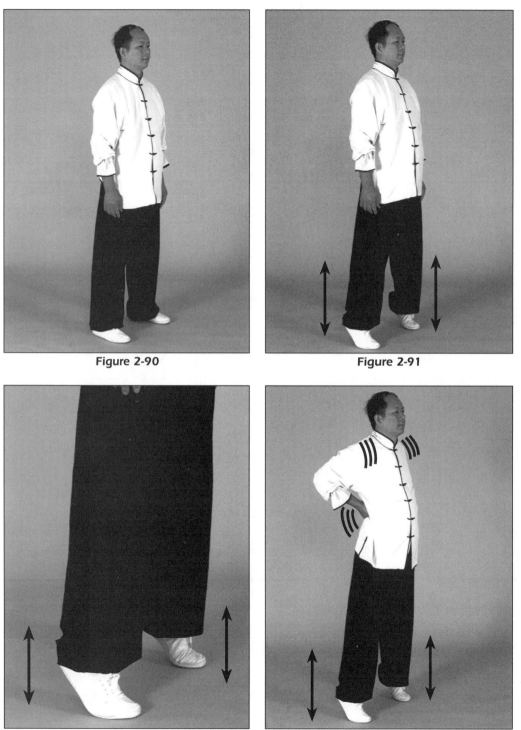

Figure 2-90

Figure 2-91

Figure 2-92

Figure 2-93

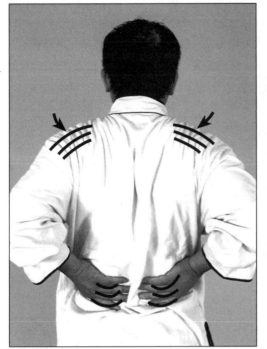

Figure 2-94

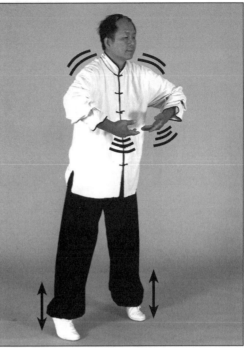

Figure 2-95

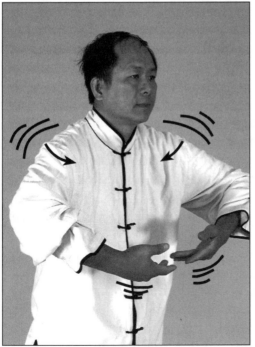

Figure 2-96

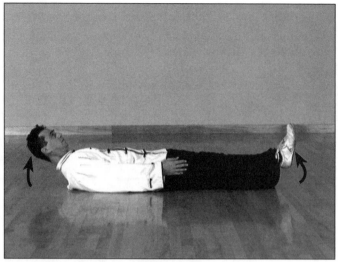

Figure 2-97

After you finish this piece, stand still, keep your mind calm, and breathe smoothly and regularly for about three minutes.

Still Wai Dan Forms

Some of the Still Wai Dan forms are very similar to Indian Yoga, which is not surprising, since China looked to India as a spiritual source for many years. The forms should be done in as relaxed a manner as possible, tensing only the muscles needed to do the posture. Place the tip of your tongue against the roof of your mouth and breathe deeply from the lower abdomen.

Form 1 (Figure 2-97). Lie on your back with your legs together and your arms at your sides. Keeping the legs straight, lift your feet about three to five inches off the floor, and at the same time lift your head and upper torso the same height. Breathe deeply and hold the position for thirty seconds. As your strength and endurance increases, you can add more time until you are able hold the posture for two or three minutes.

Form 2 (Figure 2-98). Stretch out with your head on one chair and your feet on another with the body straight. Hold the posture for thirty seconds and work up to two minutes. As you might guess, this posture is very difficult. It is almost essential to do self-hypnosis to practice it. This is the advanced form of Form 1. In Chinese martial arts training this form is called Iron Board Bridge (Tie Ban Qiao, 鐵板橋). You should not attempt this until you can hold the first form for at least two minutes.

Form 3 (Figures 2-99 and 2-100). Lie on the floor on your stomach. Bend

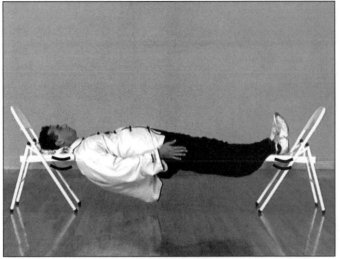

Figure 2-98

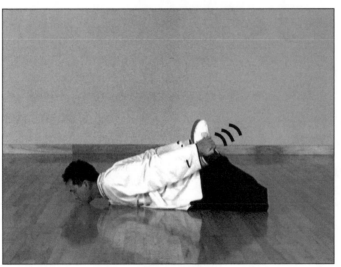

Figure 2-99

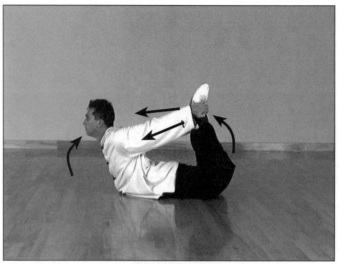

Figure 2-100

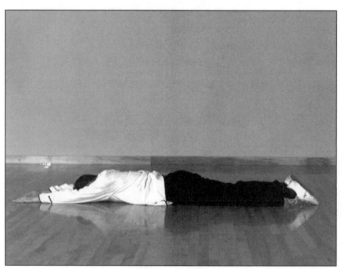

Figure 2-101

your knees and reach back and grasp the ankles or feet. Pull the feet and head toward each other as you inhale, and then relax as you exhale.

Form 4 (Figures 2-101 and 2-102). Lie on the floor on your stomach with the arms stretched forward. Simultaneously lift your upper body and your feet off the floor as you inhale, and then relax as you exhale. In Yoga, this form is called the Locust.

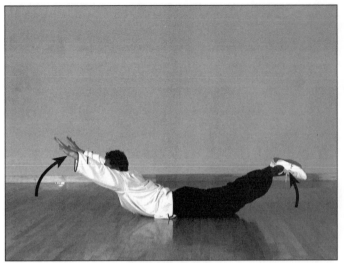

Figure 2-102

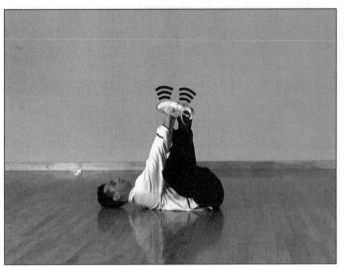

Figure 2-103

Form 5 (Figures 2-103 and 2-104). Lie on your back and grasp your feet. Slowly straighten your legs as you exhale. Return to the original position as you inhale.

Form 6 (Figure 2-105). Lie on your back with your arms by your sides. Raise your legs vertically, then continue to lift, raising the buttocks and torso off the floor. If your balance is unsteady, you may bend your elbows and use the hands

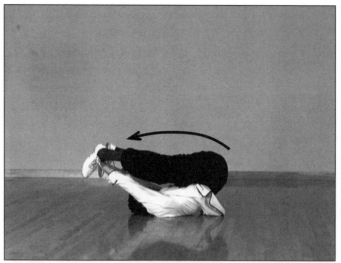

Figure 2-104

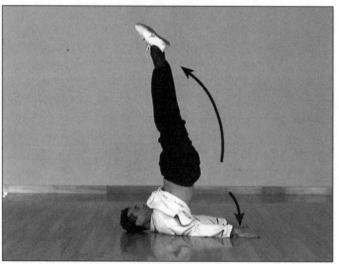

Figure 2-105

to support the trunk in a vertical position. The weight is on your shoulders and the upper arms, not on your neck. Hold this position for at least one minute, breathing slowly and deeply. This is known as the shoulder stand.

Form 7 (Figures 2-106 and 2-107). Lie on your right side, with your left knee bent so that your left knee and lower leg rest on the floor. Your right arm is straight out in front of you, your left arm is along your side. While inhaling, turn your torso so that your left shoulder and upper arm touch the floor. Your left leg remains in position. While exhaling, roll back to the starting position on the right side. Do this twenty-five times, then switch sides and repeat twenty-five times.

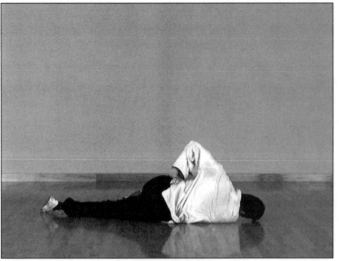

Figure 2-106

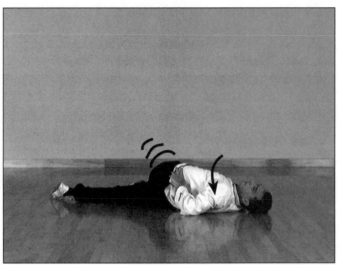

Figure 2-107

Form 8 (Figure 2-108). Assume the pushup position, resting your body weight on the fingertips. Keep your back straight. Hold for thirty seconds up to one minute.

Form 9 (Figures 2-109 and 2-110). This posture is called The Child Worships the Buddha (Tong Zi Bai Fo, 童子拜佛). Stand on one leg and extend the other straight out in front, parallel to the floor. Press your palms together in front of your chest. Hold for thirty seconds on each leg. As an advanced technique, bend your knee and lower your body on inhalation, and stand back up on exhalation.

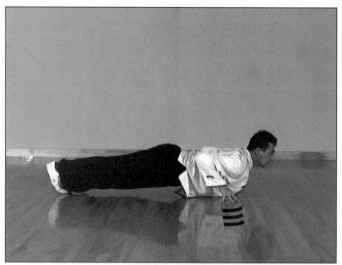

Figure 2-108

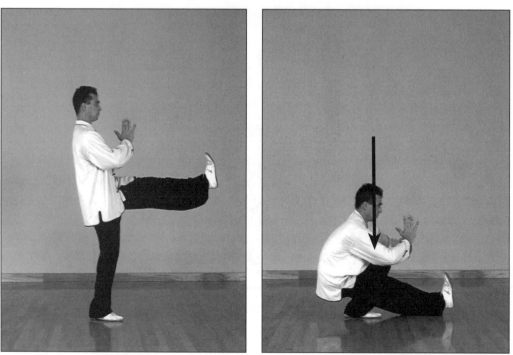

Figure 2-109   Figure 2-110

Form 10 (Figure 2-111). Stand on one leg in a half squat with the palms pressed together in front of the chest, but this time the free leg is held out in front of the body. Hold for up to three minutes on each leg.

Form 11 (Figure 2-112). Stand in a half squat with your feet shoulder width apart and parallel. Raise your arms up until the palms face the ceiling. Bend your

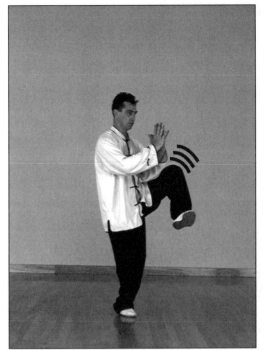

Figure 2-111

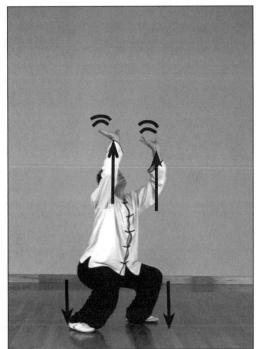

Figure 2-112

head back and look straight up. Hold for one to three minutes. This is called Tuo Tian (Holding up the Sky, 托天).

Form 12 (Figure 2-113). Stand on one leg, with the front toe of the other leg just touching the floor in front of your body. Raise your arms in a horizontal circle in front of your chest, palms facing in. Hold for three minutes on each leg.

This chapter introduces you to the principles and theory of Wai Dan exercises. Although several sets of traditional Wai Dan forms are presented, you should be able to create your own forms as long as you thoroughly understand the theory. The new forms should generate the sensation of Qi flow in the areas or sets of muscles being exercised.

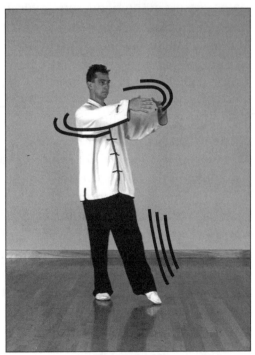

Figure 2-113

Chapter 3
Nei Dan Qigong
(Internal Elixir)
內丹氣功

3-1. Introduction

Nei Dan (pronounced "Nay Dan") literally means "internal elixir." It is a training method in which Qi is generated in the abdomen and then guided by the mind throughout the body. As was explained in chapter 1, when the muscles are exercised, Qi and blood accumulate in the area of the body being exercised. When the muscles are then relaxed, the channels open wide and allow the accumulated energy to flow from the area that was exercised and circulate throughout the body. This exercising with exterior muscles, called Wai Dan, was discussed in the previous chapter.

Nei Dan is a different process. Energy is generated in an area of the lower abdomen called the Dan Tian (下丹田) or Qihai (Co-6)(Sea of Qi, 氣海). The energy built up in the Dan Tian can be guided by the will to circulate through the two major vessels in the body, the Governing Vessel (Du Mai, 督脈) and Conception Vessel (Ren Mai, 任脈), which are centered in the back and front of the torso. This is called Small Circulation (Xiao Zhou Tian, 小周天). Eventually, energy can be directed throughout the entire body through all twelve primary Qi channels. This is called Grand Circulation (Da Zhou Tian, 大周天).

The history of Nei Dan can be traced to the very beginning of Qigong practice in China. Originally, judging from the record of Buddhist and Daoist scriptures, it was used to promote physical and spiritual health, as it still is now. The people who learned Nei Dan were scholars, Buddhist and Daoist monks, and a few common people, often sick people trying to regain their health.

In the thirteenth century, the Daoist martial style now known as Taijiquan (太極拳) was created. Taijiquan specializes in using the internal power created with Nei Dan. Though the breathing techniques used for training are different from those of the Buddhists, the principles are the same. Zhang, San-Feng (張三豐)(Figure 3-1) is credited with creating the style in the Wudang Mountain area (武當山)(Figure 3-2) located to the South of Zhong Xian (鐘縣), Hubei Province (湖北省) in China. Since that time, several other Nei Dan martial styles based on the Wudang principles have been developed, such as Baguazhang (八卦掌), Xingyiquan (形意拳), and Liu He Ba Fa (六合八法).

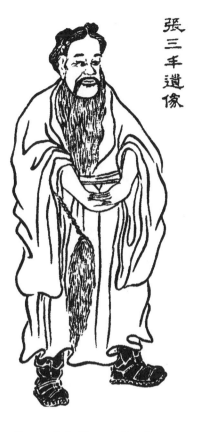

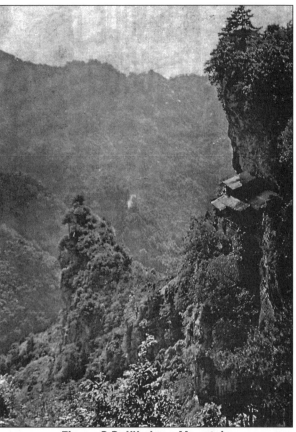

Figure 3-1. Zhang, San-Feng　　　　　**Figure 3-2. Wudang Mountain**

In the hundreds of years that have passed since then, both Shaolin Gongfu and Taijiquan have kept their respective emphasis on Wai Dan and Nei Dan secret. It was not until the late 19th century and the beginning of the 20th century, when both Shaolin Gongfu and Taijiquan were generally exposed to the Chinese public, that martial artists commonly began to practice both Nei Dan and Wai Dan.

Many other martial and non-martial styles of Wai Dan and Nei Dan were created throughout Chinese history that were popular with the Chinese people. However, most of these styles have died out, and the styles mentioned above have dominated the popular interest since the turn of the century.

Also, many non-martial systems do not use the Dan Tian as the source of Qi, but rather use some other point on the Governing or Conception Vessels, such as the solar plexus or the third eye. Energy is generated by concentrating on a selected point, not through moving the abdominal muscles. These meditation systems are outside the scope of this book and will not be discussed.

Compared with Wai Dan, Nei Dan has both advantages and disadvantages. The disadvantages are: first, with Nei Dan it takes a longer time to experience the Qi in the Dan Tian than it does to feel energy in a local area using Wai Dan. Therefore, Wai Dan Qigong can be easily applied to the martial arts in a short time, and you can see improved health and power relatively quickly. Second, Nei Dan requires more patience and a calmer mind than Wai Dan.

Finally, Nei Dan training requires instruction from a more qualified master than Wai Dan. Usually, Wai Dan training is quite straightforward once the principles and the forms are understood. However, in Nei Dan it is harder to experience Qi, so a student requires a master's advice and experienced analysis to advance step by step. Nei Dan generates a large amount of Qi and starts circulating it in the vital Governing and Conception Vessels, and it is possible that Qi can stagnate in the cavities of these vessels. Also, the generated Qi can get out of the meditator's control, go into an unexpected channel, and stay in the cavities of that channel. This Qi residue can be dangerous if the student does not know how to handle the problem. More caution and help from an experienced master is necessary in order to avoid injury.

On the other hand, Nei Dan has several advantages over Wai Dan. First, Nei Dan teaches an awareness of Qi circulation and develops this circulation more fully throughout the body, which benefits the organs more than Wai Dan. As you already know, Wai Dan circulates the Qi locally, and therefore benefits only specific organs.

Second, the Nei Dan practitioner does not have the risk of San Gong or Energy Dispersion, since Nei Dan does not build up the body's muscles except for those of the lower abdomen (the Dan Tian area), and once you practice Nei Dan for a few years, you will naturally use the Dan Tian all the time. Third, once the Nei Dan circulation is completed, the internal power it can build for martial purposes is much stronger than that of Wai Dan.

Very commonly, Chinese martial artists train both Wai Dan and Nei Dan, while non-martial artists usually practice only one or the other for health purposes.

Nei Dan can be roughly divided into Buddhist and Daoist styles. The major differences are, first, in training emphasis. Buddhists emphasize raising the Qi (Yang Qi, 養氣), in which the Qi is maintained through calmness, and is concentrated in the brain in order to reach enlightenment. In China, maintaining Qi through calmness is called Zuo Chan (坐禪) or Sitting Meditation.

In Daoist practice, however, breathing from the Dan Tian is emphasized to build up Qi and to make it stronger and stronger. This is called Lian Qi (練氣) or Strengthening the Qi. After the Qi is built up, the Daoist will circulate the Qi through the body by guiding it with his will. This is called Transporting the Qi

(Yun Qi, 運氣) or Circulating the Qi (Xing Qi, 行氣). This kind of Daoist Qigong training is commonly called Yun Gong (運功) or Xing Gong (行功), which means "the Gongfu of Qi transportation."

Second, in Qi training, Buddhists use natural breathing, in which the abdomen is drawn in when exhaling, and expanded when inhaling. The Daoists use the reverse breathing technique, in which the abdomen is drawn in when inhaling, and expanded when exhaling. It is possible that this difference stems from the Daoist use of Nei Dan in martial applications. They found it easier to express strong internal power when the Dan Tian is expanding while exhaling and sinking the Qi.

In this chapter, the next section will explain the principles of Nei Dan, and how the Qi is generated and circulated. The methods of Nei Dan training, both Buddhist and Daoist, will be introduced in section three. In section four, the secret training methods for strengthening and guiding Qi to particular areas for martial purposes will be discussed. Finally, to close the chapter, exercises and self massage techniques for after meditation will be presented in section five.

3-2. Principles of Nei Dan Qigong

As was explained before, the method in which Qi is generated in the Dan Tian or Qihai and then guided by the mind to circulate through the entire body is called Nei Dan. The location of the Dan Tian is about one and a half inches directly below the navel. The name "Dan Tian" means "Field of Elixir" and is used by Daoist meditators. The name "Qihai" is used by acupuncturists and means "Sea of Qi." The Dan Tian is considered to be the original source of a person's energy, because the embryo uses the lower abdomen to circulate its supply of nourishment and oxygen from its mother. After the baby is born, it continues to breathe with emphasis on the lower belly for several years. But gradually the focus of breathing moves higher and higher in the torso, so that by late childhood, people think of themselves as breathing with their chests, and they have lost control of their lower abdominal muscles. In Nei Dan meditation, the practitioner returns to the embryonic method of breathing; at least the focus of breathing returns to the Dan Tian because it is considered the source of Qi circulation. The Dan Tian is also called the furnace or Huo Lu (火爐)(relating meditation to Daoism's alchemical tradition) in which the fire or energy can be started.

An important Daoist classic is *Tai Xi Jing* (胎息經) or *Classic of Harmonized Embryonic Breathing*. It emphasizes the importance of the Dan Tian and regulated breathing, and recommends the nurturing of the Dan Tian as if it were an embryo. This idea is sometimes portrayed in Daoist art by a meditator with a baby over his head.

Principles From The Tai Xi Jing
胎 息 經

胎從伏氣中結，氣從有胎中息。

氣入身來爲之生，神去離形爲之死。

知神氣可以長生，固守虛無以養神氣。

神行則氣行，神住則氣住。

若欲長生，神氣相注。

心不動念，無去無來，不出不入，自然常在。

勤而行之，是眞道路。

The embryo is conceived from the hidden or undeveloped Qi.

Qi is accepted through the regulated breath of the embryo.

When Qi is present, the body may live; When Shen (Spirit) abandons the body and the embryo disperses, death will follow.

Cultivation of Shen and Qi makes long life possible. Protect and nourish the spiritual embryo to build up Shen and Qi.

When Shen moves, the Qi moves; where Shen stops, the Qi stops.

For life to flourish, spirit and energy (Shen and Qi) must harmoniously interact.

When the Xin (heart-mind) is tamed by Yi (wisdom-mind), not a thought goes or comes. (When thoughts are not going and coming), nature is free.

Intelligence in action is the only true path.

Through thousands of years of experience, Chinese meditators found that with practice they could retrain the abdominal muscles and regain a stronger flow of Qi. This exercise is called Back to Childhood (Fan Tong, 返童). Principally, when abdominal muscles are exercised, the nerves and Qi channels will accumulate the energy that has been generated by the exercise. This kind of energy generation and accumulation is called Starting the Fire or Qi Huo (起火). It is enhanced by concentrating the mind strongly on this activity. Later, it was found that in the Qi Huo exercise, the breathing must be coordinated in order to exercise the muscles efficiently and regularly. Also, this regular breath coordination helps the meditator to concentrate on the exercise. As explained in chapter 1, the mind can control Qi generation and circulation. Therefore, in meditation, you should concentrate your mind on the Dan Tian (丹田) which is called "Yi Shou Dan Tian" (意守丹田), or "The mind always stays with the Dan Tian."

Because it is a principle of Chinese meditation that the Dan Tian is the source of Qi circulation, beginning training is centered around this spot. The first thing to learn to do is to control the abdominal muscles, making them expand and contract at will, so that the lower abdomen rises and falls like a baby's. This Back to Childhood exercise can be done through frequent practice. Usually after one month of thirty minutes of daily practice, you can accomplish this control. With continued practice, the exercise will generate more and more energy. By keeping your mind concentrated on the Dan Tian, the energy will concentrate there. When the accumulated Qi is strong enough, you should be able to feel warmth in the Dan Tian.

This Back to Childhood abdominal exercise confers several benefits. First, the up and down motion of the abdominal muscles during deep breathing massages the stomach and intestines, and exercises the muscles holding the internal organs in place, and will increase their strength. This is the reason why deep breathing exercise can cure hernias, which are caused by weakness of the internal muscles. Second, exercising the abdominal muscles generates Qi not only for circulation, but also directly for the organs held and surrounded by these muscles. This Qi supply plus the increased blood circulation keeps the organs healthy. Finally, deep breathing uses the lungs to their fullest capacity, thereby strengthening and cleaning them.

If you continue to practice for another two to three weeks after the Dan Tian feels warm, you will then feel the muscles trembling or tingling. It is the accumulation of Qi in the nerves and Qi channels which causes the muscles to be out of control. This phenomenon is called Dong Chu (動觸) or Movement Sensing, in meditation. (As a matter of fact, the term "Dong Chu" is used in meditation for any kind of perceptible phenomenon caused by Qi flow, Qi redistribution, or Qi over-accumulation. The most common experiences are itching, tingling or twitching of isolated muscles, or uncontrollable shaking of the whole body). When the lower abdominal muscles begin to vibrate, it is time to guide and circulate the energy or Qi. Concentration at this moment is extremely important. You should be very calm and not get excited by the Dong Chu feeling. This phenomenon, however, does not happen to every meditator. For some, the first cycling cavities are already open and the Qi will move through them without Dong Chu happening.

Before going further, you should first understand the Qi circulation route or path. As mentioned earlier, there are two main vessels located on the front and back of the body (Figures 3-3 and 3-4). The front vessel is called the Conception

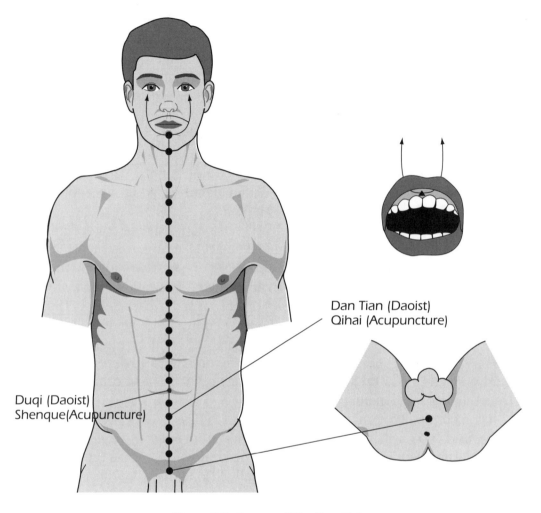

Duqi (Daoist)
Shenque(Acupuncture)

Dan Tian (Daoist)
Qihai (Acupuncture)

Figure 3-3. Course of the Ren Mai

Vessel (Ren Mai, 任脈), which contains the Yin circulation. This vessel starts from the lower lip and extends down the front center of the body to the Sea Bottom cavity (Haidi, 海底) between the scrotum or vagina and the anus. In acupuncture this cavity is called Huiyin (Co-1)(Yin Intersection, 會陰).

The vessel on the back is called the Governing Vessel (Du Mai, 督脈) and contains the Yang circulation. It starts from the Sea Bottom or Huiyin cavity and follows outside the spine, passes up the back and over the top of the head and ends at the roof of the mouth. These two vessels are not connected at the top. To connect these two vessels, you touch your tongue to the roof of your mouth.

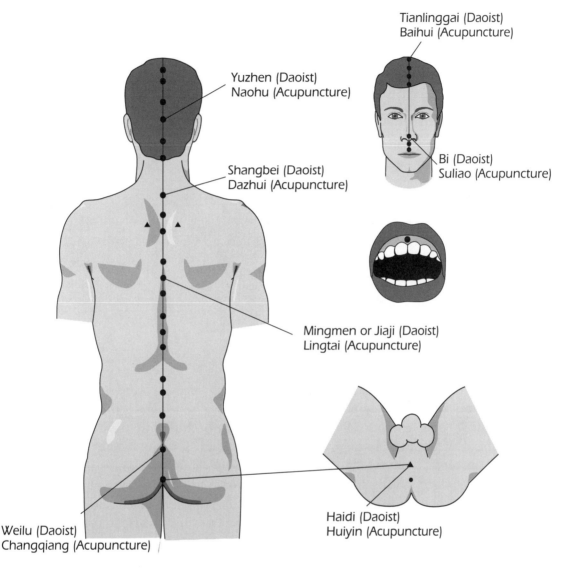

Tianlinggai (Daoist)
Baihui (Acupuncture)

Yuzhen (Daoist)
Naohu (Acupuncture)

Bi (Daoist)
Suliao (Acupuncture)

Shangbei (Daoist)
Dazhui (Acupuncture)

Mingmen or Jiaji (Daoist)
Lingtai (Acupuncture)

Haidi (Daoist)
Huiyin (Acupuncture)

Weilu (Daoist)
Changqiang (Acupuncture)

Figure 3-4. Course of the Du Mai

Then the Yin and Yang vessels are connected and the circuit is complete. This tongue touch is called Da Qiao (搭橋) or Building the Bridge.

The tongue acts like a switch in an electrical circuit. If this bridge is not built, the circuit is not complete and the Qi circulation will be incomplete. Therefore, if you meditate either in Wai Dan or in Nei Dan, keep your tongue touching the roof of the mouth all the time. Of course, we all frequently touch

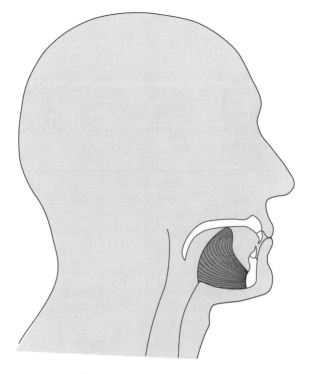

Figure 3-5. Tongue Position

the roofs of our mouths with our tongues during everyday activities. However, in meditation, a continuous circuit is important. The tongue should be relaxed and lightly touch the center of the roof of the mouth (Figure 3-5). If the tongue is tight, it will result in stagnation of the Qi flow. Also, the tongue should not touch the teeth, which will not connect the bridge efficiently, and may make you feel sleepy. On the other hand, the tongue should not be stretched to touch the back of the roof of the mouth. This will make the tongue muscles tight and sore and will also stagnate the Qi flow. If you create the tongue bridge properly, saliva will be secreted during meditation. Swallow this saliva to keep your throat moist. The place under the tongue where the saliva is produced is called the Tian Chi (Heaven's Pond, 天池), or Long Quan (Dragon Spring, 龍泉).

When you can circulate the Qi through the two major vessels, you have completed Small Circulation (Xiao Zhou Tian, 小周天). Usually, if you meditate three times a day for half an hour with the right method, you can complete this circulation in ninety days. However, it is not uncommon to take longer. The time needed to accomplish Small Circulation depends on the degree to which you can concentrate, relax, understand the techniques and principles, and feel the

Qi flow. It is very important that you do not try to hurry the process, because this will make the circulation worse and might be dangerous.

You should understand that Qi is and always has been circulating all the time in your body. However, the Qi circulation can become stagnant or slow. This is because there are many knots in the vessels and Qi channels, where the channels are narrower or harder to penetrate. Usually, these knots are located at cavities. The main purpose of Nei Dan meditation is to open or widen these knots and enable the Qi to flow without stagnation. When Qi is stagnant and does not flow smoothly, you will soon feel sick and the related organ will become weakened. When the Qi channels are open, the arteries will also be open and will allow the blood to flow smoothly. This is because the arteries usually follow the Qi channels. For this reason, meditation is often able to alleviate high blood pressure.

In Nei Dan Small Circulation, there are three cavities or knots that are harder to pass through than the others, and might cause difficulties (Figure 3-4). These are called the San Guan, 三關) or Three Gates.

The first cavity is called Weilu (Tailbone, 尾閭) by the Daoists and Changqiang (Gv-1)(Long Strength, 長強) by the acupuncturists. It is located at the tailbone.

The second cavity is called Jiaji (Squeezing Spine, 夾脊) by Daoists. Jiaji is called Lingtai (Gv-10)(Spirit's Platform, 靈台) by acupuncturists and Mingmen (Life's Door, 命門) by Chinese martial artists. The martial artists use the name Life's Door because a strike to this point can cause a heart attack and kill an opponent. (There is also a cavity called Mingmen (Gv-4) by acupuncturists which belongs to the Governing vessel).

The last cavity is called Yuzhen (Jade Pillow, 玉枕) by Daoists and Naohu (Gv-17)(Brain's Household, 腦戶) by acupuncturists, and is located at the base of the skull. Further explanation of these three cavities will be given in the next section. These cavities offer the greatest resistance to increased Qi flow, and so are the three major milestones for judging progress in achieving Small Circulation.

While controlling the Qi as it circulates, you should be able to feel a flow of energy, following the guidance of your mind. However, you can also feel the back muscles beside the vessel expanding and tensing. This feeling of expansion will not happen when the Qi goes above the Jade Pillow cavity at the back of the head. Instead, you will feel only the energy or Qi flow, since there is no thick muscle on the head to feel. The usual feeling of Qi flow on the head is local numbness or tickling, as though insects were brushing the skull.

During meditation, you may find your body naturally swinging or rocking forward and backward. You may also feel a muscle jump or contract by itself. These are all symptoms of Dong Chu caused by Qi redistribution. All of this is normal, and you have nothing to be alarmed about.

Once you have accomplished Small Circulation, you can then try to master Grand Circulation, which circulates energy to the entire body through the twelve Qi channels. Usually, you will either concentrate only on your arms or only on your legs first, and then go to the other limbs. However, it is also common, once you complete Small Circulation, to practice guiding the Qi to the upper and lower limbs simultaneously and to imagine Qi expanding from the two main vessels.

In the next section, both Buddhist and Daoist meditation methods will be discussed. Before you start meditation, read this and the following sections repeatedly, until you are sure you understand them. If you are interested in knowing more about Nei Dan meditation, please refer to the books: *The Root of Chinese Qigong* and *Muscle/Tendon Changing* and *Marrow/Brain Washing Chi Kung*, available from YMAA Publication Center.

3-3. Nei Dan Meditation Training

Small Circulation (Xiao Zhou Tian) 小周天

Meditation Breathing. The first and most important step for effective meditation is proper breathing. There are two basic methods in use in Chinese meditation: Daoist and Buddhist.

Daoist breathing, also known as Reverse Breathing (Fan Hu Xi, 反呼吸), is used to prepare the Qi for circulation, and its proper development is crucial. In Daoist breathing the normal movement of the lower abdomen is reversed during inhalation and exhalation. Instead of expanding when inhaling, the Daoist contracts, and vice versa (Figure 3-6). Never hold your breath or force the process. Inhale through the nose slowly, keeping the flow smooth and easy, and contract and lift the lower abdomen up behind the navel. When the lungs are filled, exhale gently.

Inhalation is considered Yin and exhalation is considered Yang. They must operate together like the Yin-Yang symbol, one becoming the other smoothly and effortlessly in a fluid circular motion. As exhalation occurs, slowly push out the Dan Tian or lower abdomen. The area of the Dan Tian is where the Qi is generated and accumulated in order to start Small Circulation. Because of this, the muscles around the Dan Tian must be trained so that they can sufficiently contract and expand while you inhale and exhale. At first, expanding the lower

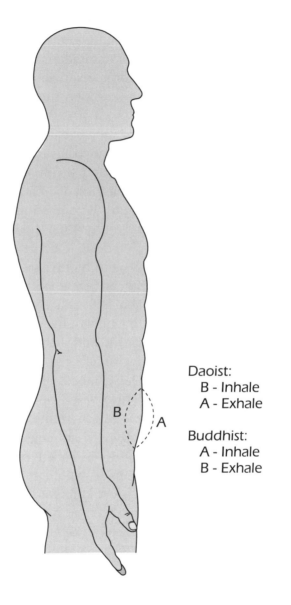

Daoist:
  B - Inhale
  A - Exhale

Buddhist:
  A - Inhale
  B - Exhale

Figure 3-6. Abdominal Motion During Breathing

abdomen while exhaling may be difficult; but with practice the muscles learn to expand more and more until the entire lower abdomen expands upon exhalation from the navel to the pubic bone. Do not force the Dan Tian to expand, but work gently until success is achieved.

This whole process of Daoist breathing is a form of deep breathing, not because the breathing is heavy, but because it works the lungs to near capacity. While many people who engage in strenuous exercise breathe hard, they do not necessarily breathe deeply. Deep breathing causes the internal organs to vibrate in rhythm with the breath, which stimulates and exercises them. The organs would not receive this type of internal exercise without deep breathing. Many forms of strenuous exercise only condition the external muscles, while doing very little for the vital organs.

In the Buddhist breathing method, the movement of the abdomen is the opposite of the Daoist. When you inhale, expand your lower abdomen, and when you exhale, contract it (Figure 3-6). This kind of breathing is called Normal Breathing (Zhen Hu Xi, 正呼吸). It is the same kind of breathing a singer practices.

Both methods use the same principle of Qi generation. The main difference is that the coordination of the abdominal motion and the breathing is opposite. In fact, many meditators can use either method, and switch very easily.

Meditation and Qi Circulation. Once you can breathe adequately according to the Daoist and Buddhist methods, you can take up sitting meditation to begin the process of Qi circulation. The first goal is to achieve a calm mind while concentrating on deep breathing. You create a type of hypnotic state to do this. You should stay at this stage until you can expand and withdraw your Dan Tian while breathing with no conscious effort, and without your attention wandering.

When the muscles around the Dan Tian can be easily controlled, the process of breathing acts like a pump to start a fire, which is Qi production, in the furnace of the Dan Tian. This whole process of generating and accumulating Qi in the Dan Tian is called Lower Level Breathing (Xia Ceng Qi, 下層氣), while simple exhalation and inhalation in the lungs is called Upper Level Breathing (Shang Ceng Qi, 上層氣). One system aims at building Qi as energy, while the other aims at building up Qi as air. The over-abundant Qi in the Dan Tian will cause the abdominal area in most people to twitch and feel warm. The pump (the deep breathing) has thus caused a fire (an accumulation of Qi) in the Dan Tian area. When this occurs, the Qi is ready to burst out of the Dan Tian and travel into another cavity.

In order to insure that the accumulated Qi passes into the correct cavity, the sitting posture must be correct (legs crossed). When the Qi is ready to burst from the Dan Tian, it must not be allowed to travel into the legs. By having the legs properly crossed, the Qi is partially blocked. If the Qi does go downward, it may stagnate in some of the cavities. If you are a novice meditator, this is dangerous, since you do not have enough experience with or understanding

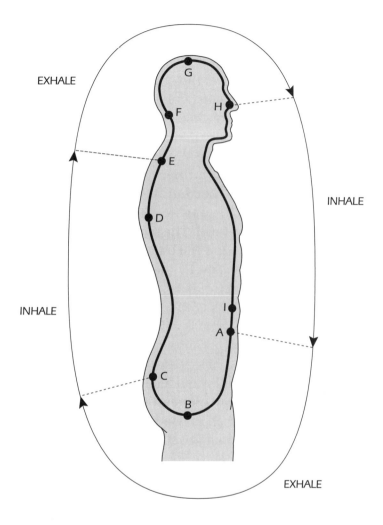

Figure 3-7. Breathing and Qi Circulation—Two Breath Cycle

of controlling Qi with your will. This Qi residue in the cavities will later affect the Qi circulation in your legs, and might, in extreme cases, cause paralysis. When Qi goes into an undesired Qi channel and causes problems, it is called Zou Huo (走火) or Fire Deviation. Therefore, during any serious meditation session in which you attempt to circulate Qi, your legs must be crossed. Only after Small Circulation has been totally achieved and you are attempting Grand Circulation is it permissible to uncross the legs.

In order to correctly initiate Small Circulation, the Qi must pass into the Weilu cavity, located in the tailbone. Thus, the Qi passes from the Dan Tian down through the groin area, called the Bottom of the Sea (Haidi, 海底), and into the tailbone. The Qi does pass through other acupuncture cavities on the way to the Weilu (Figure 3-4), but the Weilu will offer the greatest resistance because the bone structure narrows the channel.

During meditation your mind must guide the Qi consciously throughout its circulation. Without the mind consciously leading the circulation of Qi, there will be no consistent or smooth circulation. It sometimes happens that the Qi will pass from the Dan Tian into the Weilu without conscious effort, but the mind must actively guide the Qi for further results. Starting from the Dan Tian, the mind remains calm and fully concentrated only on guiding the Qi past the Weilu. This process must never be pushed. Simply keep the mind on the next cavity and let the Qi get there by itself. The requirement of concentration is one of the reasons why simple relaxation will only promote local circulation. For the larger circuits, the Qi must be guided by the will.

In Daoist breathing, the secret of bringing the Qi to the Weilu is to tighten the anus gently while inhaling. This is called Bi Gang (Close the Anus, 閉肛) in meditation. When exhaling, the anus is relaxed and Qi is guided to the Weilu. This is called Song Gang (Relax the Anus, 鬆肛). This coordination should be done even after Small Circulation has been completed.

After the Qi has been successfully guided to the Weilu, it moves up the spine to the next major obstacle, the Jiaji (Squeezing Spine, 夾脊) or Mingmen (Life's Door, 命門). This point is located on the back directly behind the heart between the spinous processes of the sixth and seventh thoracic vertebrae (Figure 3-4). As mentioned earlier, this same cavity is called Lingtai (Spirit's Platform, 靈台) in acupuncture. When Qi flows to this area, it will usually cause the heart to beat faster, which can interfere with concentration. To lose concentration at this point might result in the Qi dispersing in this area, which can cause a cold sweat, tensing of the nerves, and rapid breathing. If the Qi remains in the surrounding area, it will stagnate the Qi flow in that area, and disturb the heart function. However, if you relax, concentrate on the cavity, and remain calm, there is usually little resistance to the Qi flow here.

Once the Qi passes the Jiaji, the last major obstacle on the spine is called the Yuzhen (玉枕), or Jade Pillow by meditators, and Naohu (腦戶) by acupuncturists. This cavity is located at the base of the skull on top of the occipital bone (Figure 3-4). Because of the skull structure, the channel is constricted here. If the energy does not pass smoothly through, it may pass into other channels on the head or into the brain. If this happens, you may experience headaches or fever-ish thinking.

Once the Qi enters the head, the sensation of Qi circulation is different from that of the circulation on the back. Circulation on the back causes the large spinal muscles to tense, and it is easy to feel. However, when the Qi enters the head, where the muscle layer is very thin, you will feel no muscle tension. What you will feel is a tingling sensation, like insects walking on your scalp, that will travel over the top of your head to the front of your face.

The above three major cavities are called the Three Gates or San Guan (三關) in Chinese meditation.

After the Qi passes through the Yuzhen, your mind guides the Qi up over the top of the head, down the middle of the face and chest, and finally back to the Dan Tian, where the cycle starts over. Once you have achieved a complete Small Circulation cycle, then the whole process is done continuously. Achieving Small Circulation requires three sessions of meditation each day for a period of nine-ty or more days. Grand Circulation may take years to achieve.

Up to this point, little has been said about breathing during Qi circulation. The cyclic movement of Qi must coordinate with deep breathing. Figure 3-7 shows the basic pattern of Daoist meditation, which consists of guiding the Qi through one cycle of Small Circulation during two sets of breaths (Table 3-1 lists the names of the important points and their corresponding abbreviations on Figures 3-7 to 3-9). This is the cycle that beginners should attempt.

To begin, during the first inhalation your mind guides the Qi from the nose to the Dan Tian. Next, exhale and guide the Qi from the Dan Tian to the Weilu. Then, inhale and lead the Qi up to the point at the top of the shoulders, called the Shangbei (上背) or Dazhui (Gv-14)(大椎)(see Table 3-1). Finally, exhale and guide the Qi over your head to your nose to complete one cycle. Continue cir-culating the Qi, one cycle every two breaths.

After you are proficient with the two-breath cycle, you can circulate Qi in a one-breath cycle. This cycle is the basis for using Qi as the energy source in the martial arts. Figure 3-8 shows the one-breath cycle. You guide the Qi to the tail-bone while exhaling, and then to the nose while inhaling.

Some beginning meditators say they cannot feel the Qi flow, while others say they feel it is stopped at a particular point. The response to both of these comments is to continue doing the cycle. At first, it will be mostly your imagi-nation and not much Qi, but with perseverance the flow will become stronger, more complete, and more perceptible. Remember, the Qi is always flowing or you would not be alive. Since Qi follows the mind, keeping your attention

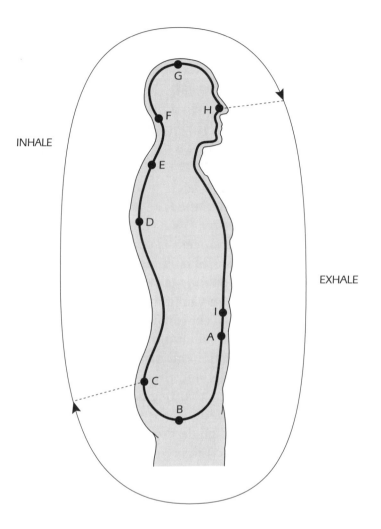

Figure 3-8. Breathing and Qi Circulation—One Breath Cycle

moving will keep the Qi flowing through the channels and gradually open the constrictions.

Advanced students can try reversing the current of Qi in Small Circulation so that the Qi travels up the chest, over the top of the head, down the back, and then to the Dan Tian. In reverse circulation, the transition points of Qi between inhalation and exhalation remain the same. Thus, inhale and guide the Qi from the Dan Tian to the nose; next, exhale and guide the Qi over the head to the Shangbei. The next step is to inhale and guide the Qi to the tailbone (Weilu).

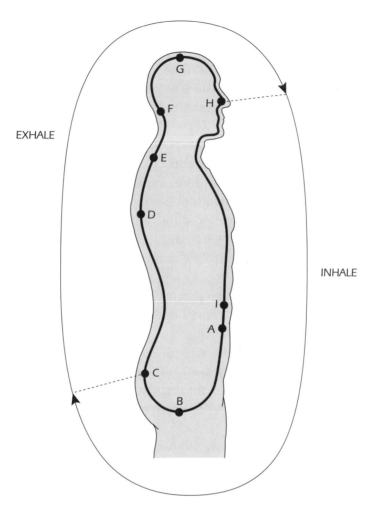

Figure 3-9. Breathing and Qi Circulation—Buddhist Method

Table 3-1

Point	Daoist Name	Acupuncture Name	Location
A	Dan Tian (下丹田)	Qihai (氣海)	One and half inches below the navel
B	Haidi (海底)	Huiyin (會陰)	Pelvic floor
C	Weilu (尾閭)	Changqiang (長強)	Tailbone
D	Mingmen (命門)	Lingtai (靈台)	On the spine behind the heart
E	Shangbei (上背)	Dazhui (大椎)	Upper back
F	Yuzhen (玉枕)	Naohu (腦戶)	Base of the skull
G	Tianlinggai (天靈蓋)	Baihui (百會)	Crown of the skull
H	Bi (鼻)	Suliao (素髎)	Nose
I	Duqi (肚臍)	Shenque (神闕)	Navel

Finally, exhale and guide the Qi to the Dan Tian. The one-breath cycle follows the same principle. This reversed circulation can help heal injuries and can clear blockages that the regular circulation has difficulty passing through.

Included with the one-breath cycle described above is the Buddhist system of Qi circulation (Figure 3-9). The Buddhist meditator inhales and guides Qi from the nose, down the chest through the groin to the tailbone. Then he exhales and guides the Qi up the spine, then over the head to the nose. Buddhists can also reverse the direction of the cycle. Remember that in the Buddhist method, the Dan Tian expands during inhalation and contracts during exhalation.

There are also methods of meditation that do not use the Dan Tian as the source of Qi. Some systems use the solar plexus, the forehead, or other points, and generate Qi through concentration alone, without breath coordination.

Novice Meditators. If you are coming to meditation seriously for the first time, you should not attempt to circulate Qi from the very start. The primary goal of the beginner must be to train the muscles around the Dan Tian so that the Daoist method of breathing is easy and natural. The training of the muscles is achieved through the preliminary practice of reverse breathing. Once your muscles have been adequately trained and your mind sufficiently calmed, you may then attempt to circulate the Qi.

Pre-meditation Warm-up. Before meditation, you should spend three to five minutes calming your mind. Once your mind is calm you can begin concentrated meditation with better results. Calming your mind before meditation may be thought of as a warm-up exercise. For more experienced meditators, the warm-up takes less time.

Posture. Two common cross-legged postures appropriate for meditation are shown in Figures 3-10 and 3-11. Pick the one that is most comfortable for you. In any posture, your back should be straight without being bolt upright; do not slouch. It is easiest to sit on a cushion about two to five inches thick with the knees or feet on the floor at a lower level. This helps to keep the back straight without strain.

If your legs become numb while sitting, uncross them and relax. With continued practice you will be able to sit comfortably for longer and longer periods. This usually takes several weeks. Sitting cross-legged restricts the normal flow of blood and Qi, and the body needs to learn to adjust to the new position.

In both sitting positions your hands should be held at the Dan Tian, one on top of the other, with the tips of the thumbs touching. This position helps you to feel your breathing as you expand the Dan Tian, and to coordinate deep breathing and Qi circulation.

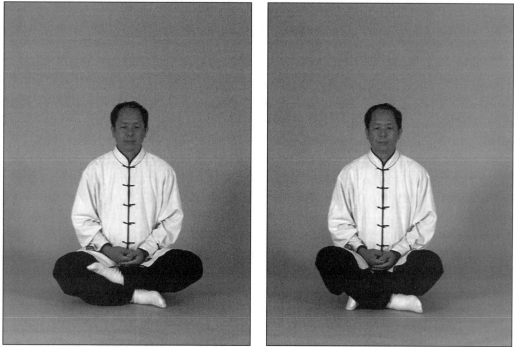

Figure 3-10   Figure 3-11

Geographical Positioning. While meditating, you should face east in the morning and face south at night. This common practice was most likely established because experienced meditators discovered that their Qi circulation was more fluid when they faced east in the morning. This may be because the rotation of the earth enhances the flow of Qi slightly, and also because of the energy of the early morning sun. Meditators face south at night because the earth's magnetic field originates from the South Pole. If you face the south, you obtain energy nourishment from the earth.

Time of Meditation. Ideally, you should meditate three times a day for one half hour at a time. The best times to practice are fifteen minutes before sunrise (facing east), one to two hours after lunch (facing east), and one half hour before going to sleep (facing south). With this schedule you can, if you remain calm and concentrated, achieve Small Circulation in about three months.

These three times are the best because the morning and evening meditations take advantage of the changing of the body's energy from Yin to Yang, and vice versa. The afternoon is the best time to calm the mind and cool the body's excess Yang state.

If you can only meditate twice a day, skip the afternoon session. If only once, then meditate in either the morning or evening. Reducing the number of sessions means taking longer to achieve Small Circulation. Do not be discouraged by this. Instead, enjoy what you are learning and doing, proceed with care, and you will achieve your goal.

Thoughts. During meditation your mind should focus on the Dan Tian and on the Qi circulation. The whole purpose of meditation is lost if your mind wanders. You must achieve a relaxed hypnotic trance; this is easily done by concentrating on the rhythmic pattern of your breathing. If your attention does stray, or if thoughts arise, simply return your attention to your breathing.

If you have too many day-to-day worries bothering you during meditation, do not meditate and do not attempt to circulate Qi. Instead, breathe deeply for relaxation. Attempting to circulate Qi while emotionally agitated can only harm you.

Position of the Tongue, Teeth, and Eyes. During meditation, your tongue should lightly touch the roof of your mouth near its center. This touch creates a bridge between Yin and Yang and allows the Qi to circulate in a continuous path around the body. Take care that your tongue is neither too far forward nor too far back—both will hinder meditation. Too far forward causes sleepiness, too far backward hinders relaxation, and the tension obstructs the Qi flow.

The tongue bridge also allows saliva to accumulate in your mouth. Swallow this saliva occasionally to keep your throat from getting dry. In addition, your teeth should touch lightly.

You can keep your eyes closed or half open during meditation. Do not let yourself become sleepy if your eyes are closed.

The Mechanics of Meditation.

Cautions—Here are a few general rules that will prevent you from causing yourself injury, and will help you speed the process of meditation.

1. Don't smoke. Because meditation involves deep breathing, your lungs must be able to function adequately.
2. Don't drink to excess. Too much alcohol will hurt the nervous system and hinder Qi circulation. Naturally, you should not drink just before meditating. Alcohol can affect your neutral judgment.
3. Wash before meditation. However, you should wait at least fifteen minutes so that your body temperature resumes its normal state. This will help relax your mind.
4. Wear loose, comfortable clothing, especially around the waist.

5. Meditate in a well ventilated area.

6. Men should avoid sex twenty-four hours before and after meditation.

7. During their periods, women should not concentrate on the Dan Tian, but instead on the solar plexus.

8. Meditate in a quiet place where you will not be disturbed.

9. Wait at least half an hour, and preferably one or two hours, after eating to meditate.

10. Do not meditate if you are worried or ill.

11. Never hold your breath.

12. Always remain relaxed while meditating.

13. Always concentrate on the Dan Tian and on the Qi flow.

14. If you repeatedly feel bad or get strongly unpleasant reactions during meditation, stop. Do not proceed without the guidance of a qualified and experienced meditation master.

Common Problems:

Numb legs: This problem affects nearly everyone who begins sitting meditation, especially those who are unused to sitting cross-legged. It is caused by a reduced flow of blood and Qi to the legs. The problem gradually goes away by itself. Until then, you should stop meditation when the numbness disturbs your concentration. Stretch out your legs to open the channels and use acupressure or massage on the arches of the feet to speed recovery. As soon as feeling returns, resume meditation.

Cavity pain: Some meditators experience pain in the tailbone, at the kidneys, at the Life Door (Mingmen, Gv-4, 命門), or at the joints of the inner thighs when Qi circulation reaches these spots. It is caused by increased pressure at that point, often because of Qi stagnation. The sensation is normal and can be relieved through relaxation. Ordinarily, this kind of pain will only last two or three days, or until the circulation has passed that spot.

Headache: This is caused by tension, worry, fatigue or when circulation first reaches the head. If it is caused by tension or worry, stop meditating until you calm down. If you are too tired to concentrate, it would be better to take a nap. If it is the result of excess Qi flow to your head, simply relax more and pay attention to your breathing and to the Dan Tian. Some of the pain can be relieved by using the massages described in the next section.

Backache: Backaches can be caused either by improper posture or by a residue of stagnant Qi. If your posture is too stiffly erect, or if you slump, there will be too much tension in the back muscles and a backache will result. To assume a comfortable posture, sit up very straight, stretching upward as far as possible, then relax without bending forward.

A residue of stagnant Qi is sometimes dangerous and should be treated with heavy massage. See the next section for a description of effective massage techniques.

Drowsiness: Drowsiness is a result of being too tired, in which case you should stop meditating. Take a nap until you feel alert enough to meditate again.

Sweating: If sweating is a result of the environment, that is, if the place where you meditate is too hot or too humid, try to change it. If the sweating is not a result of environmental factors, there are two kinds of sweating—hot and cold. Cold sweats may indicate an injury to one of the cavities in the path of circulation. Consult a meditation master who can help to clear the obstruction. Hot sweats are usually caused by circulating the Qi without concentrating, and go away with improved concentration and relaxation.

Grand Circulation (Da Zhou Tian, 大周天)

After you can circulate your Qi at will in the two main vessels (i.e. Small Circulation), you can begin the practice of Grand Circulation, in which you circulate the Qi generated at the Dan Tian through all the Qi channels in your body.

By this time you should be able to feel the Qi generating and flowing around your body through the Governing and Conception vessels. With this experience as a basis, you should be able to accomplish Grand Circulation easily and safely through mental control of the Qi.

To circulate Qi to your arms and hands using Grand Circulation, you can either sit in a chair or stand up. In Grand Circulation training, your whole body should be relaxed. Hold your arms out in front of your body, with the elbows slightly bent. Hold your hands so the palms face forward and your fingers point up. In this exercise, the thumb and little finger of each hand should be slightly tightened by pulling them back in order to restrict the Qi flow and force it to the palms.

As you inhale, bring the Qi from the tailbone up your back to the top of the shoulders (Figure 3-12). Inhaling also prepares the Qi on the front of the body for a new cycle. As you exhale, guide the Qi not over your head, but into your arms. At the same time that the Qi flows into your arms, your Dan Tian expands,

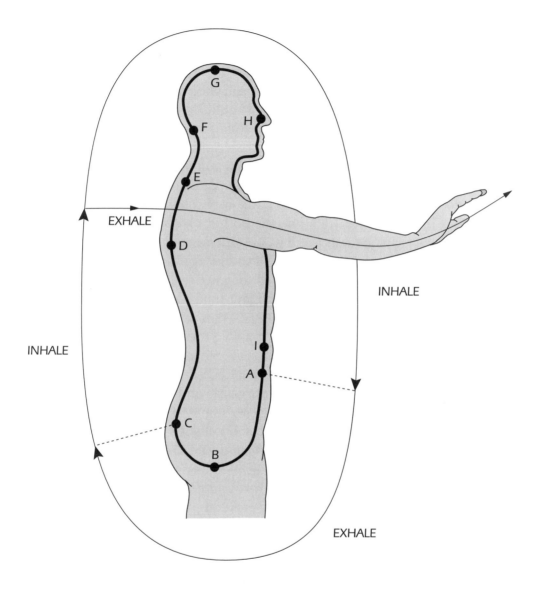

Figure 3-12. Grand Circulation

starting a new cycle by moving the new Qi into the tailbone. When you inhale again, guide the Qi to the upper back while preparing for a new cycle on the front of the body. Thus, the Qi cycle is a one way path, in that it does not travel in a complete circle, but in a line that ends in the hands. This cycle is repeated continuously until you can feel the Qi flow to the center of the palms, to a cavity called the Laogong (P-8, 勞宮) cavity. (In fact, the Qi does circulate back to the Dan Tian, but concentrating on a one-way flow pushes the circulation out to the hands sooner and more strongly.)

When the Qi approaches your palms, you should be able to sense it and feel the warmth. After this is achieved, you should then try to guide Qi to the fingertips. There are many methods of practicing circulation to the upper limbs. You should refer to the next section for descriptions.

To circulate Qi to the lower limbs, a common method is to lie on your back and relax the leg muscles, which opens the Qi channels. Inhale and contract your abdomen, then exhale and guide the Qi through the legs to the Bubbling Well point (Yongquan)(K-1, 湧泉) on the bottoms of your feet (see Figure 3-13). Normally the Qi channels in the legs are open wider than those in the arms. Consequently, it is easier to circulate Qi to the legs than to the arms. When the Qi approaches the bottoms of your feet, they will feel warm and numb, and this feeling may persist for several days the first time you experience it.

Some teachers recommend following certain paths to and from the feet and hands. This is not really necessary. If you lead the Qi into your feet and hands, it will find its own way there, and in time will fill your limbs, moving through all the channels, both Jing (經) and Luo (絡). Keep in mind, too, that leading (i.e., guiding the Qi with your mind) is always gentle and relaxed.

Because the leg channels are open, it is sometimes possible to circulate Qi while standing, even though the muscles are slightly tense. This is the reason that Taijiquan practitioners can accomplish Grand Circulation through the slow motion exercise of Taiji.

After you can circulate Qi to the arms and legs, you have achieved Grand Circulation within your body. This can take six months to achieve, or many years, depending on you and the time you have available for practice.

Beyond Grand Circulation, you can develop the ability to expand the Qi to the arms and legs simultaneously (Four Gates Breathing, 四心呼吸); to expand the Qi in the form of a ball larger than the body (Skin Breathing, 體息、膚息); and to take in Qi from outside the body, or direct the Qi at will to specific parts of the body, such as the joints, fingertips, or the area of an injury.

If you learn to transport Qi beyond your body or to take in Qi from outside, then you may be able to use Qigong to cure illness and injuries involving Qi disturbances. However, this should not be attempted without training from an experienced instructor. To take outside, disturbed Qi, called evil Qi (Xie Qi,

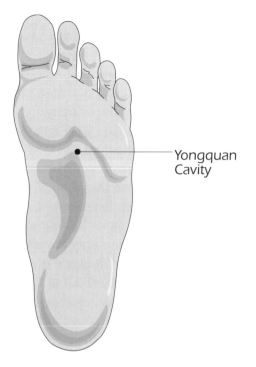

Yongquan
Cavity

Figure 3-13. Yongquan Cavity

邪氣) into your body without knowing how to get rid of it is dangerous. By the same token, if you extend your own Qi into another body without knowing the proper stopping point, you run the risk of Qi exhaustion.

3-4. Qi Enhancement and Transport Training

Once you have accomplished Grand Circulation, you can begin to practice advanced methods to make your Qi stronger, more focused, and more controlled by your will. Even though you can start this Qi enhancement after accomplishing Small Circulation, the enhancement will be easier and more efficient if you wait until the completion of Grand Circulation.

The first training method of Qi Enhancement and Transport is called Lian Qi (Train the Qi, 練氣) or Chong Qi(Filling Qi, 充氣). The main purpose of this training is to fill the Dan Tian with Qi, so that when Qi is accumulated there the abdomen is resilient like a balloon and can endure or resist a strong attack. As the Qi gets stronger and stronger in the Dan Tian, the Qi flow in the body also gets stronger and stronger.

The training method of Chong Qi is simply to blow out a candle. Start two feet away, and increase the distance as you are able. Tighten your lips to form a very small opening, and blow air out through this opening slowly and steadily, imagining that the stream of air is directed at the flame and does not spread out at all. Blow as long as possible without straining. While blowing, imagine that Qi is expanding and accumulating in the Dan Tian. When you can blow the candle out easily from a distance of two feet, move the candle further away and continue. Practice five to ten minutes daily.

A method of Lian Qi, called Kuo Qi (Expanding Qi, 闊氣), is to extend the Qi in a ball outward from the surface of the body. To do this, exhale and imagine that your Qi is expanding out from your body in all directions, forming a globe, and the center of the globe is the Dan Tian. When you become proficient at this, you will feel as if your body has disappeared, that you are transparent, and that you are a ball of Qi that gets smaller and smaller when you inhale and expands when you exhale. This exercise not only enhances the symmetrical movement of Qi, but also enables the Qi to reach every cell of the body simultaneously. This is known as Body Breathing (Ti Xi, 體息) or Skin Breathing (Fu Xi, 膚息).

After Qi development is at a fairly strong level, you can learn to focus or concentrate your Qi at some small area of the body. This kind of training is called Yun Qi (運氣) or Transporting the Qi. The main use of Yun Qi training is in the martial arts, where the Qi is concentrated in the palms for attack. Also, Qi can be transported to a specific area to resist a blow or punch. This latter Yun Qi practice is part of Iron Shirt (Tie Bu Shan, 鐵布衫) or Golden Bell Cover (Jin Zhong Zhao, 金鐘罩) training. See chapter 5 for more information.

Several training methods are described below. The first task is to learn to focus the Qi in the palms. It is a slow process in the beginning, but with practice it will happen instantaneously.

1. The first form is called Gong Shou (Arcing the Arms, 拱手)(Figure 3-14), in which the arms form a circle in front of your body with the fingertips close together, but not touching. Gong Shou can be done either sitting or standing. When you exhale, guide the Qi to the arms and fingertips and imagine the energy exchanging at the fingers, from one hand to the other. The Qi should flow to the hands from both arms at the same time, circling in both directions simultaneously.

2. In the second form, hold your hands as if you are holding a basketball in front of your chest. Your elbows should not bend too much, because the Qi flow will stagnate at the elbow area (Figures 3-15 through 3-17). Your mind should guide the Qi through the air from both palms, exchanging energy as in (1) above. The palms should move about continuously as though rotating an imaginary ball to gain

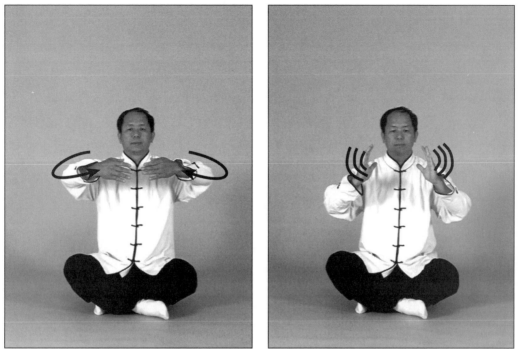

Figure 3-14   Figure 3-15

the feeling of the smooth Qi flow. Often, Taijiquan practitioners perform this exercise while holding an actual ball to develop the feeling of a smooth, circular flow. However, the imaginary ball works well, so a real ball is not necessary.

3. In the third form, lightly touch your palms together in front of your chest (Figure 3-18), and exchange the Qi from one palm to the other while exhaling.

4. The fourth form is a finger touch, which is more advanced than the palm touch. Touch your fingertips together lightly in front of your chest (Figure 3-19), and exchange energy between your hands while exhaling.

5. The fifth form is a horizontal circling Qi flow called Wave Hands Like Clouds (Yun Shou, 雲手) in Taijiquan. Hold your right forearm at chest level parallel to the ground with the palm facing inward in front of the breast bone, elbow slightly lower than the rest of the arm. Hold the left hand palm down at waist level in front of your body (Figure 3-20). Exhale and turn your torso smoothly to the right as far as possible while directing the Qi to the palms (Figure 3-21). Exchange the hands while inhaling (Figure 3-22) and turn to the other side while exhaling (Figure 3-23). This sequence should be repeated continuously in a flowing rhythm.

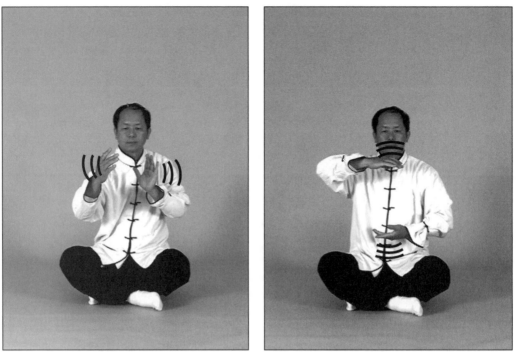

Figure 3-16   Figure 3-17

6. The sixth form is sinking palm training. When inhaling, lift both your arms with the palms facing each other (Figure 3-24) and when exhaling, imagine pressing down on a resistant object while using only a little muscle tension (Figure 3-25). This will lead the Qi to the palms or to the edges of your hands. When inhaling, release the tension.

7. The seventh form is palm pushing training. There are three directions of pushing palm training.

a. Push forward when exhaling and move inward when inhaling (Figures 3-26 and 3-27).

b. Push out to the sides when exhaling, and from the outside in when inhaling (Figures 3-28 and 3-29).

c. Up and down with hands exchanging. When extending upward and downward, exhale. When moving your hands toward the center, inhale (Figures 3-30 and 3-31).

d. Up and down with both hands at once. When pushing upward, exhale, and when moving downward, inhale (Figures 3-32 and 3-33).

When you practice any one of these seven forms, with each exhalation imagine pushing with your palms against a resistant object and guiding the Qi to

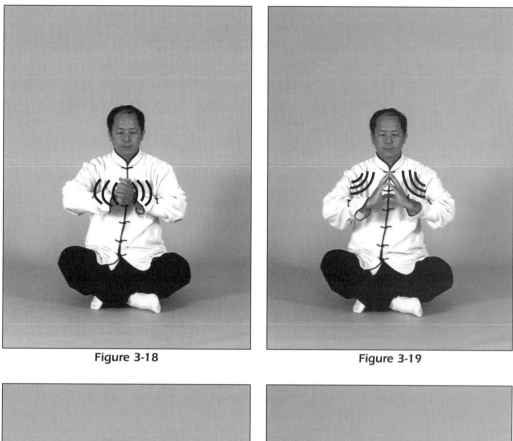

Figure 3-18

Figure 3-19

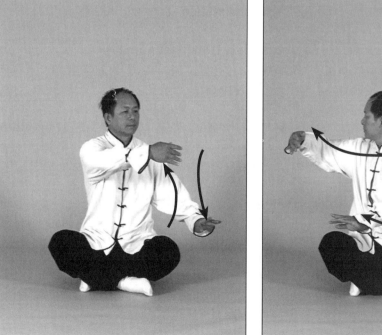

Figure 3-20

Figure 3-21

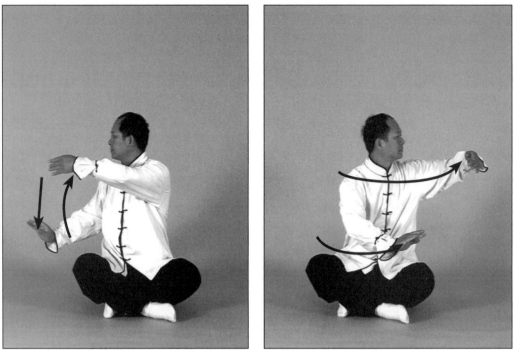

| Figure 3-22 | Figure 3-23 |

your palms with slight muscular tension. Before you try these exercises, first push a wall to experience the feeling of resistance. This will help you to better imagine your push.

Other than the above seven forms of Qi transport and concentration training, there are two other common ways of practicing, both of which use a candle. The first way is the secret sword Qi transport (Figure 3-34). To do this, hold both hands in the secret sword form. Your index and middle fingers point out, and the rest of your fingers are closed. Point one of your hands at a candle flame. Begin with the fingertips one to two inches away. While exhaling, transport the Qi to the flame to make the flame move. If you practice faithfully, you will be rewarded by being able to make the flame bend away from you.

The second way of training is again to make the candle flame bend, but this time with the palm held five to ten inches away (Figure 3-35). This is similar to the secret sword form, except that this time the Qi is directed out from the palm instead of the fingers. Either way, the hand not being pointed toward the flame should be kept in the same form and held in front of the abdomen for symmetry. Make sure when you do these exercises that your breath is directed away from the candle, and that only the Qi flow moves the flame.

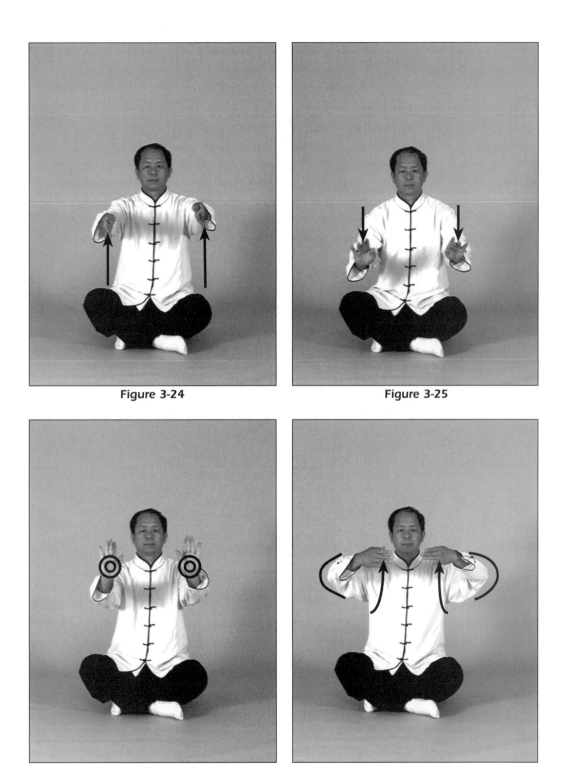

Figure 3-24

Figure 3-25

Figure 3-26

Figure 3-27

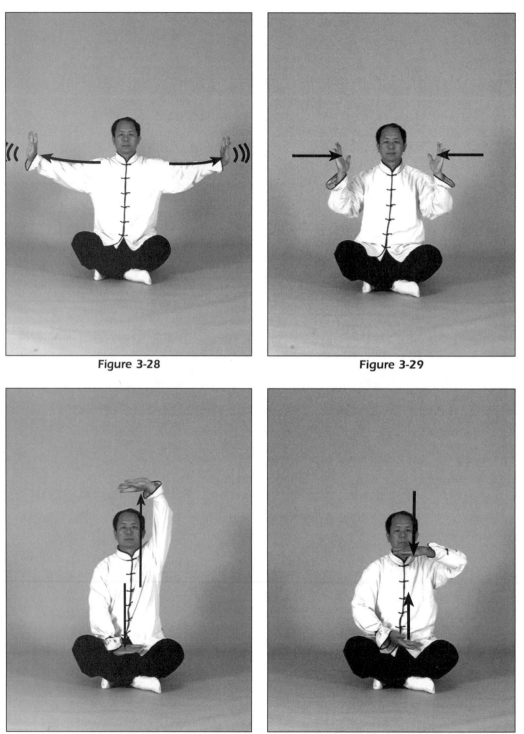

Figure 3-28

Figure 3-29

Figure 3-30

Figure 3-31

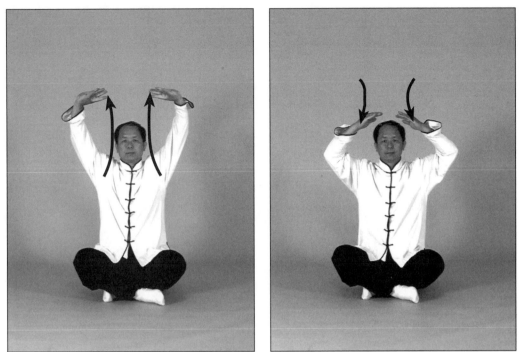

Figure 3-32   Figure 3-33

3-5. Massage and Exercises after Meditation

After meditation or Qi transport training, you should massage yourself and do some loosening up exercises. The main purpose of massage is to loosen and relax the muscles on the Qi pathways. This can help you to clear your mind, and can also help to eliminate any Qi residue that might remain in certain cavities. This residue of stagnant Qi, if left in the cavities, can affect normal Qi circulation and cause muscle and cavity pain. If a partner is available, it is best to massage each other, because it is easier to relax that way. Furthermore, a partner can massage the pathways on your back, which is difficult to do by yourself.

Massage

Head. Begin with the face. Rub the ridge of the brow starting at the nose (Figure 3-36) and move your hands up and across the forehead until your fingers pass the temple (Figure 3-37). Next put your hands under the eyes (Figure 3-38) and rub across the cheeks. Third, put your thumbs in front of the ears (Figure 3-39) and move the thumbs down to the chin. For the top of the head, place your fingers one inch off the centerline of the skull (Figure 3-40). Move the scalp back and forth lightly. Reset the fingers along the same lines, but toward

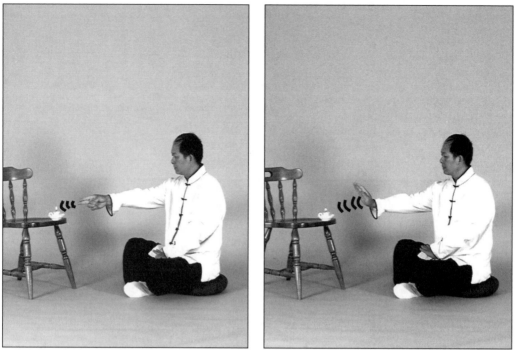

Figure 3-34   Figure 3-35

the back, and gently rub again. Keep moving your fingers back along the head and massaging until you reach the back of the skull. The last place to rub in the head area is the neck. Place your thumbs at the base of the skull and rub downward with the hands (Figure 3-41).

Hands. Rub the palms together (Figure 3-42) then rub the center of the palm with your thumb (Figure 3-43). In the center of the palm is Laogong cavity (P-8, 勞宮) which lies on the pericardium channel. By massaging this cavity, the heart is gently stimulated.

Kidneys. Make fists with both hands and place the knuckles or the back sides of your palms on your back at the kidneys. Rub in a circular motion (Figure 3-44).

Knees. During meditation your knees may become stiff and absorb cold air through the pores. To warm them up and relieve stiffness, use an open hand to rub around the whole joint (Figure 3-45).

Feet. Rub the center of the bottom of your foot with the thumb (Figure 3-46). This stimulates the kidneys via the Yongquan cavity (K-1, 湧泉). You may then massage the entire bottom of the foot.

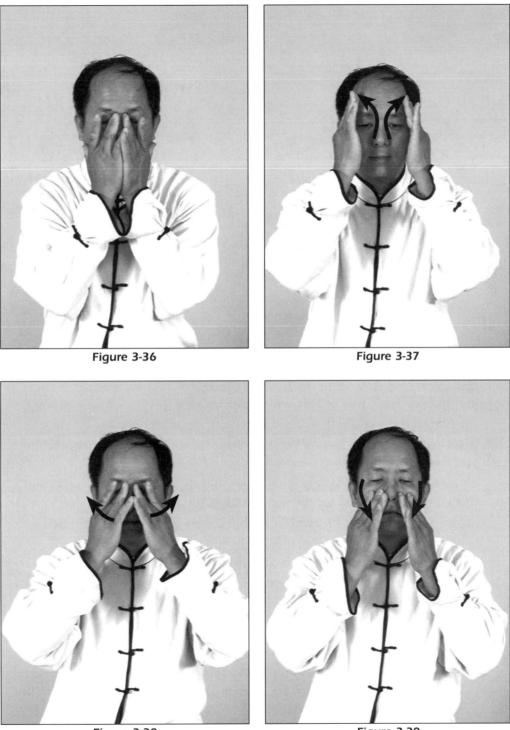

Figure 3-36

Figure 3-37

Figure 3-38

Figure 3-39

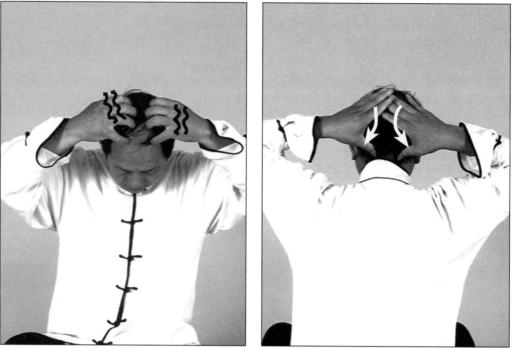

| Figure 3-40 | Figure 3-41 |

General Exercises After Meditation

1. Rotate your head by slowly turning it from side to side without moving the rest of the body (Figure 3-47).

2. Rotate your back by slowly twisting your torso from side to side while you remain in the sitting position (Figure 3-48).

3. Stretch your chest by clasping your hands behind your back and thrusting the chest as far forward as possible (Figure 3-49).

4. Rotate your shoulders forward and backward (Figures 3-50 and 3-51).

5. Lock your fingers with the palms facing out, then stretch your arms out in front of your chest (Figure 3-52) and over your head (Figure 3-53).

6. Stretch your legs by grasping your feet and straightening your legs (Figure 3-54).

Beating the Heaven Drum (Ming Tian Gu, 鳴天鼓)

The Ming Tian Gu exercise is very important in Qigong training, and should always be practiced after meditation. It helps you to awaken completely from

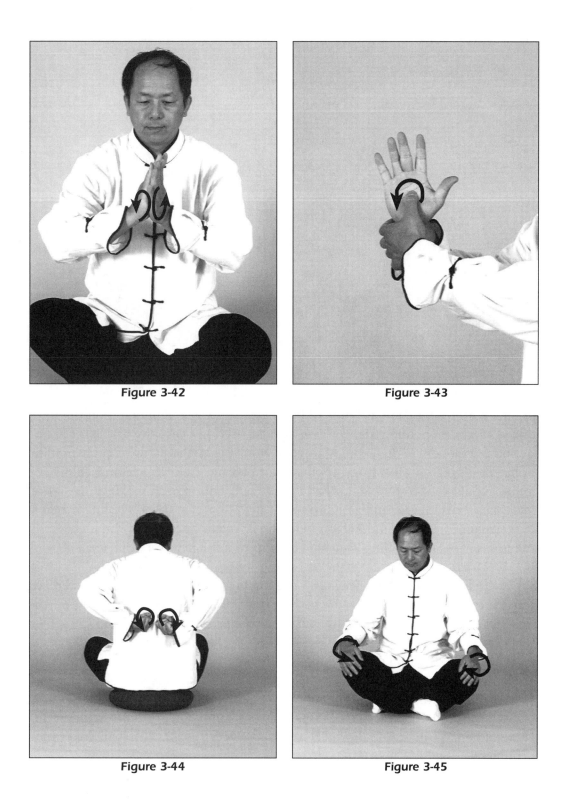

Figure 3-42

Figure 3-43

Figure 3-44

Figure 3-45

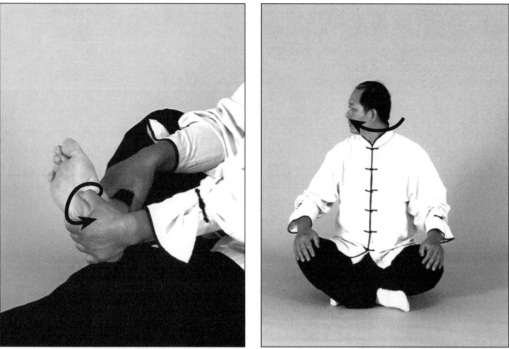

Figure 3-46   Figure 3-47

the meditative state, and it helps to flush away any Qi accumulated in the head during meditation. Ming Tian Gu can also be used in everyday life. After a long period of concentration, it helps to clear your mind, the same as after meditation. The Daoists found that tapping the head not only clears and calms the mind, but also improves memory and judgment. This is because the stimulation increases the supply of nutrients to the brain. Ming Tian Gu is helpful for relieving headaches, especially tension headaches, again because of the increase in the flow of Qi. Finally, Ming Tian Gu can improve the health of the scalp if practiced regularly, and prevent hair loss and graying.

There are two common ways to beat the heaven drum. In the first exercise, tap the top and back of your head, or crown (Figure 3-55), especially on the acupuncture points (Figure 3-56), with your fingertips. When you tap the crown this way, the resulting stimulation to the Qi channels and nervous system increases Qi and blood circulation in the head.

In the second exercise, cover your ears with your palms and place the middle fingers on the Jade Pillow cavity area (Yuzhen, 玉枕)(under the external occipital protuberance)(Figure 3-57). Put your index fingers on the middle fingers, and snap them down to hit your head (Figure 3-58). This will generate a drumming sound in the brain cavity.

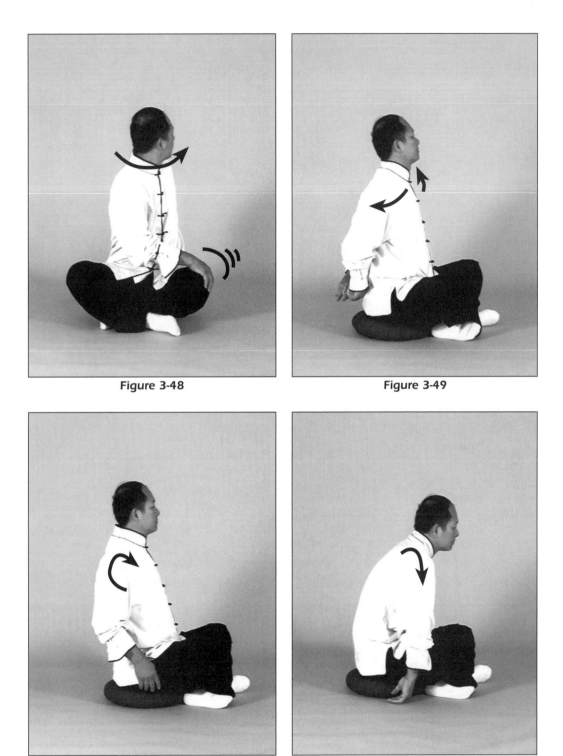

Figure 3-48

Figure 3-49

Figure 3-50

Figure 3-51

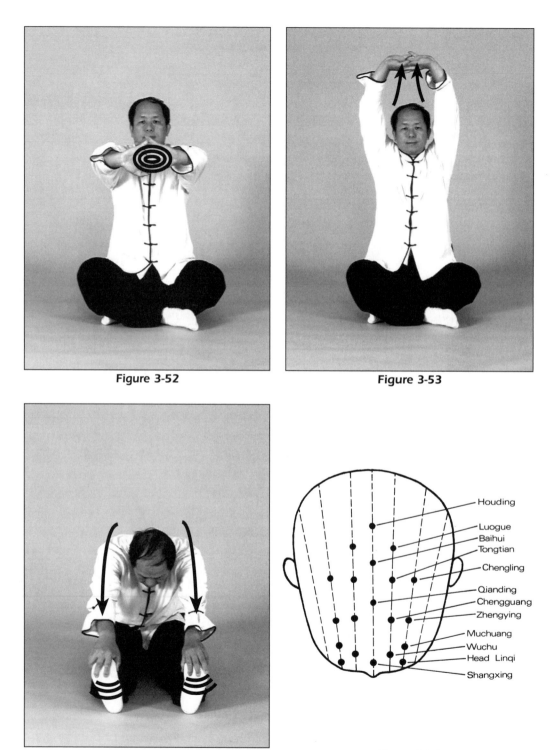

Figure 3-52

Figure 3-53

Figure 3-54

Figure 3-55

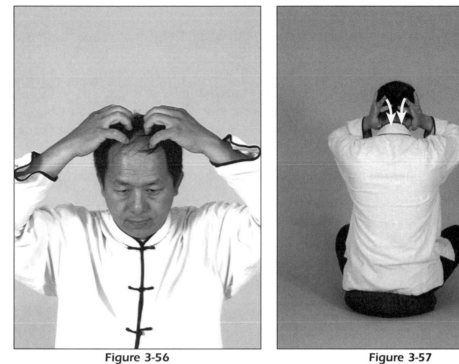

Figure 3-56   Figure 3-57

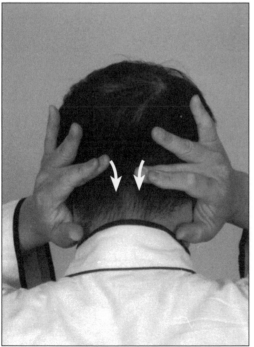

Figure 3-58

Knocking the Teeth (Kou Chi) 扣齒

Kou Chi is commonly used together with Ming Tian Gu after meditation. It consists of simply biting vigorously (but not too hard) about fifty times. The knocking causes reverberations in the skull, which helps to clear the mind, and also promotes the health of the teeth by stimulating their roots.

If you are interested in knowing more about Ming Tian Gu, Kou Chi, and other medical Qigong exercises, please refer to the book: *Eight Simple Qigong Exercises for Health*, available from YMAA Publication Center.

Chapter 4
Qigong and Health

氣功與健康

4-1. Introduction

Qigong was originally researched and developed by the Chinese to promote good health. For more than four thousand years they have investigated human Qi circulation, its relationship with the seasons, weather, and time of day. The Chinese found that Qi is closely related to altitude, location, food, emotional states, and even the sounds a person makes. They have done much research into methods of maintaining good Qi circulation. These methods can roughly be divided into the categories of maintenance and healing. The first category specifies methods that are used to maintain a person's health, and minimize the degeneration of the organs in order to increase the lifespan. The second specifies techniques that are used to cure illness.

In maintenance Qigong, the Qi is built up either by Wai Dan or Nei Dan, and then guided by the mind to circulate through the entire body. According to acupuncture theory, smooth Qi circulation is the key to health. When Qi is stagnant in a channel, the related organ will be weakened and will degenerate. Maintenance Qigong prevents stagnation.

In healing Qigong, techniques are applied to patients to control the Qi circulation and gradually heal the disordered internal organs, or cure an external injury. The methods most generally used include acupuncture, massage, and rubbing. Although Wai Dan and Nei Dan are primarily used to maintain smooth, abundant Qi circulation, advanced meditators sometimes use Wai Dan and Nei Dan to eliminate internal bruises and Qi stagnation caused by injuries. Recently, it has been found in China that Wai Dan and Nei Dan can be used to cure some cancers.

From acupuncture theory we know that the Qi channels are distributed throughout the entire body. These channels are closely related to the internal organs and are also related and connected to each other. All these channels have terminals at the hands, feet or head. Because of this, the Chinese doctor looks at a patient's face, tongue, and eyes, and feels the pulses in the wrist to understand the severity of the illness and its prognosis.

For the same reason, Qi circulation can be stimulated by massaging the ears, hands, and feet. These techniques are known as reflexology, and have proven very effective.

In this chapter, the diagnostic techniques of Chinese physicians will be briefly described in section two. The theory and techniques of acupuncture will be discussed in section three. If you want more information about diagnosis and acupuncture, please refer to specialized texts on these subjects. In section four, the theory and techniques of massage will be introduced, and skin rubbing methods will also be summarized.

4-2. Chinese Diagnosis

When you are sick, Qi circulation is irregular or abnormal. It has too much Yin or too much Yang. Because all Qi channels are connected to the surface of the body, stagnant or abnormal Qi flow will cause signs to show on the skin. Also, when you are sick, the sounds you make when speaking, coughing, or breathing are different than when you are healthy. Therefore, Chinese doctors examine a patient's skin, particularly the forehead, eyes, ears, and tongue. They also pay close attention to the person's sounds. In addition, they ask a number of questions about daily habits, hobbies, and feelings to understand the background of the illness. Finally, the doctor feels the pulses and probes special spots on the body to further check the condition of specific channels. Thus, Chinese diagnosis is divided into four principal categories: 1. Looking (Wang Zhen, 望診); 2. Listening and Smelling (Wen Zhen, 聞診); 3. Asking (Wen Zhen, 問診); and 4. Palpation (Qie Zhen, 切診).

Obviously, Chinese medicine takes a somewhat different approach to diagnosis than Western medicine. Chinese doctors treat the body as a whole, analyzing the cause of the illness from the patient's appearance and behavior. Often what the Chinese physician considers important clues or causes are viewed by the Western doctor as symptomatic or irrelevant, and vice versa.

Next, we will briefly discuss the above four Chinese diagnostic techniques:

Looking (Wang Zhen, 望診)

The doctor looks at the spirit and inspects the color of the patient.

General Appearance. The doctor examines the facial expression, muscle tone, posture, and general spirit of the patient.

Skin Color. The doctor examines the skin color of the injured area, if the problem is externally visible, like a bruise or pulled muscle. The doctor also examines the skin color of the face (Figure 4-1). Since some channels are connected to the face, its color reveals what organs are disordered or out of balance.

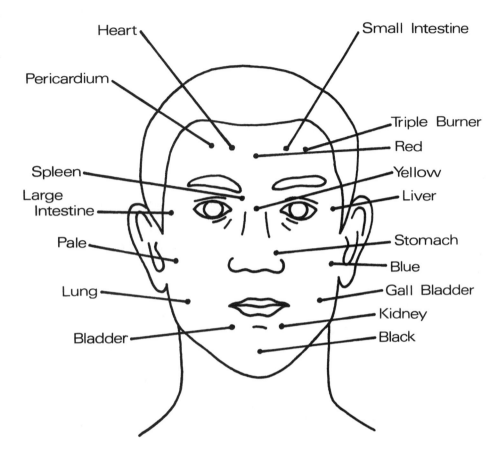

Figure 4-1. Diagnosis by Inspecting the Color of the Face

Tongue. The tongue is closely connected through Qi channels to the heart, kidney, stomach, liver, gall bladder, lungs, and spleen (Figure 4-2). In making a diagnosis, the Chinese doctor will check the shape, fur, color, and the body of the tongue to determine the condition of the organs.

Eyes. From the appearance of the eyes the doctor can tell the liver condition. For example, when the eyes are red, it means the liver has too much Yang. Also, black spots on the whites of the eyes (Figure 4-3), can tell of problems with the Qi circulation, degeneration of organs, or stagnancy due to an old injury.

Hair. The condition of the hair can indicate the health of the kidneys and the blood. For example, thin, dry hair indicates deficient kidney Qi or weak blood.

Lips and Gums. The color of the lips and their relative dryness indicates if the Qi is deficient or exhausted. Red, swollen, or bleeding gums can be caused by stomach fire. Pale, swollen gums and loose teeth might be a symptom of deficient kidneys.

Listening and Smelling (Wen Zhen, 聞診)

The doctor listens to the patient's breathing, mode of speech, and cough. For example, a dry, hacking cough is caused by dry heat in the lungs.

The doctor smells the odor of the patient's breath and excrement. For example, in the case of diseases caused by excessive heat, the various secretions and excretions of the body have a heavy, foul odor, while in diseases caused by excessive cold, they smell more like rotten fish.

Asking (Wen Zhen, 問診)

This is one of the most important sources of a successful diagnosis. The questions usually cover the patient's past medical history, present condition, habits and life style. Traditionally, there are ten subjects a Chinese doctor will focus on in this interview. They are:

1. Chills and fever
2. Head and body
3. Perspiration
4. Diet and appetite
5. Urine and stool
6. Chest and abdomen
7. Eyes and ears
8. Sleep
9. Medical history
10. Bearing and living habits

Palpation (Qie Zhen, 切診)

There are three major forms of palpation (touching or feeling) in Chinese medicine:

1. The palpation of areas which feel painful, hot, swollen, etc. to determine the nature of the problem. For example, swelling and heat indicates there is too much Yang in the area.

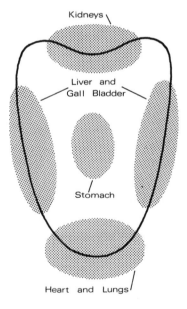

Figure 4-2. Diagnosis by Inspecting the Condition of Tongue

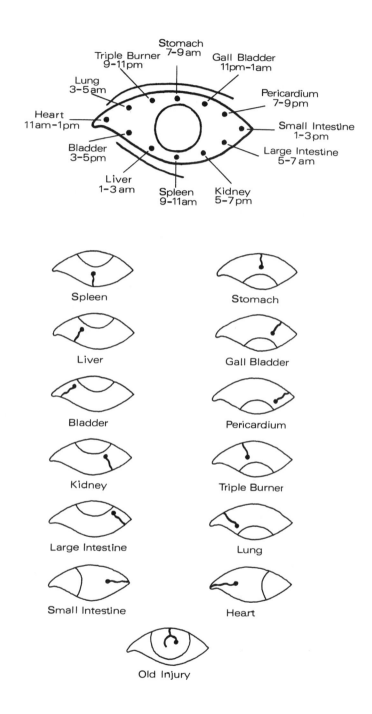

Figure 4-3. Diagnosis by Inspecting the Black Spot in the Eyes

2. The palpation of specific acupuncture points on the front and back of the trunk. For example, if the doctor senses a collapsed feeling, or the point is sore to touch, this indicates the possibility of disease in the organ with which the point is associated.

3. The palpation of pulse: Traditionally, the radial area pulse on the wrist (Figure 4-4) is the principal site for pulse diagnosis. Although the pulse is specially related to the lungs and controlled by the heart, it refers the condition of all organs (Table 4-1). The doctor checks the following: the depth (floating or submerged), the pace (slow or fast), the length (long or short), the strength (weak or strong), and the quality (slippery, rough, wiry, tight, huge, fine, or irregular). Usually it takes several years and hundreds of cases to become expert in the palpation of pulse.

Recently, inspection of skin eruptions on the ears has been used in Chinese diagnosis. A number of sites have been found on the ear (Figure 4-5) which become spontaneously tender or otherwise react to disease or injury somewhere in the body. Stimulation of these ear points in turn exerts certain therapeutic effects on those parts of the body with which they are associated. Moreover, many Western diagnostic methods, such as X-rays, have also been adopted in coordination with Chinese diagnosis.

This section serves only as a brief introduction to Chinese medical diagnosis. Interested readers should refer to books about Chinese medicine for more information.

Table 4-1

The Palpation of Pulse

Left Hand	Organs
Rear	Kidney Yin
Middle	Liver
Front	Heart

Right Hand	Organs
Rear	Kidney Yang
Middle	Spleen
Front	Lungs

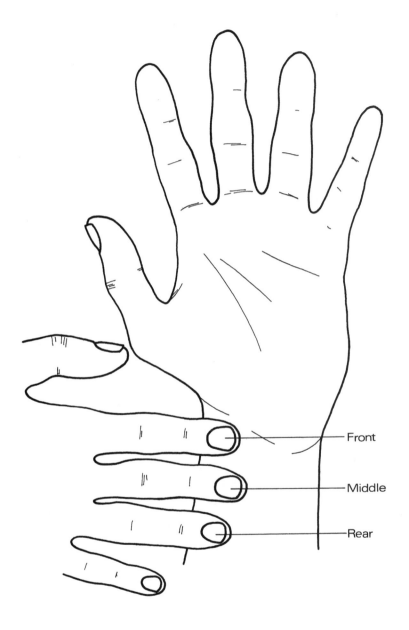

Figure 4-4. Locations Used for Pulse Palpation

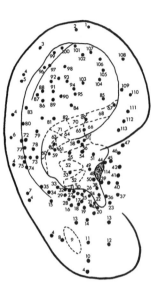

1. Pt. Ear Apex
2. Pt. Tonsilla
3. Pt. Ganyang
4. Helix
5. Pt. Ganyang
6. Pt. Tonsilla
7. Pt. Tonsilla
8. Pt. Auris Interna
9. Pt. Facies and Bucca
10. Pt. Tonsilla
11. Pt. Oculus
12. Anesthetic points for tooth extraction
13. Pt. upper and lower Mandible
14. Pt. Lingua
15. Pt. Nephritis
16. Pt. Vertex
17. Pt. Taiyang
18. Pt. Hypophysis
19. Pt. Emphysema
20. Pt. Oculus (Astigmatism)
21. Pt. Frons
22. Pt. Hormone
23. Pt. Oculus (Glaucoma)
24. Pt. Subcortex
25. Pt. Pingchuan
26. Pt. Testis
27. Pt. Excitation
28. Pt. Nervus
29. Pt. Occiput
30. Pt. Encephalon
31. Pt. Vertigo
32. Pt. Brain Stem
33. Pt. Collum
34. Pt. Glandula Thyroidea
35. Pt. Clavicula
36. Pt. Endocrine
37. Pt. Hypertension
38. Pt. Bronchiectasis
39. Pt. Glandula Suprarenalis
40. Pt. Hunger
42. Pt. Thirsty
43. Pt. Ovarium
44. Pt. Tragic Apex
45. Pt. Pharyngo Larynx
46. Pt. Cor (Xinzang)
47. Pt. Auris Externa
48. Pt. Sanjiao
49. Pt. Bronchus
50. Pt. Glandula Parotis
51. Pt. Cardia
52. Pt. Pulmo
53. Pt. Cor
54. Pt. Ventriculum
55. Pt. Ptosis
56. Pt. Fulcram
57. Pt. Diaphragm
58. Pt. Mid-crus Helicis
59. Pt. Jisong
60. Pt. Lien
61. Pt. Uterine Appendages
62. Pt. Lowering Blood Pressure
63. Pt. Duodenum
64. Pt. Intestinum tenue
65. Pt. Appendix Vermiformis
66. Pt. Intestinum Crassum
67. Prostata
68. Pt. Vesica Urinaria
69. Pt. Ureter
70. Pt. Ren
71. Pt. Pancreas and Gall Bladder
72. Pt Shoulder
73. Pt. Glandula Mammaria
74. Pt. Art. Humeri
75. Pt. Thorax Externa
76. Pt. Shoulder Ache
77. Pt. Subaxilla
78. Pt. Thorax
79. Pt. Abdomen
80. Pt. Appendix Vermiformis
81. Pt. Lumbago
82. Pt. Appendix Vermiformis
83. Pt. Cubitus
84. Pt. Nates
85. Pt. N. Ischiadicus
86. Abdomen
87. Pt. Lower Abdomen
88. Pt. Genu
89. Pt. Fever
90. Pt. Cavum Pelvis
91. Pt. Popliteal Fossa
92. Pt. Sura (Calf)
93. Pt. Shenmen
94. Pt. Hepatitus
95. Pt. Guguan
96. Pt. Carpus
97. Pt. Allergy
98. Pt. Art. Coxae
99. Pt. Digitas Manus
100. Pt. Appendix Vermiformis
101. Pt. Digitum Pedis
102. Pt. Malleolus
103. Pt. Asthma
104. Pt. Os
105. Pt. Uterus
106. Pt. Esophagus
107. Pt. Calx
108. Pt. Hemorrhoid
109. Pt. N. Sympathetica
110. Pt. Organa Genitalia Externa
111. Pt. Urethra
112. Pt. Anus
113. Pt. Lower Rectum
114. Pt. Nasus Internus

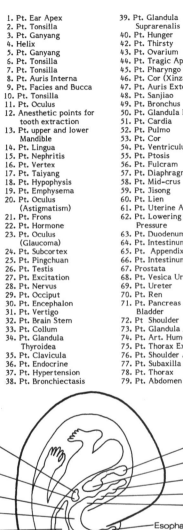
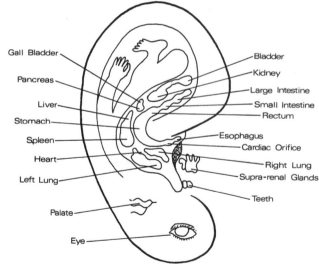

Figure 4-5. Acupuncture Points in the Ear

4-3. Acupuncture

In this section, we will discuss how acupuncture is used, and why it works. Since Qigong exercises and Qi circulation theory are based on the results of acupuncture research, this summary will help you understand the theory of Qigong exercises.

In order to understand acupuncture, you should know what Jing (經) and Luo (絡) are. Then you should understand their function in the body, and their relationship to health.

Jing and Luo are the Qi channels that connect the inside of the body to the surface of the body, and connect the internal organs to each other. They correspond with the vascular system with its arteries, veins, and capillaries. Jing are the primary Qi channels which distribute Qi in the body. Usually, Jing are found under a thick layer of muscle, and so are protected from external influence, the same way the arteries and main nerves are. There are twelve Jing which connect the internal organs with the rest of the body.

Luo are the minor or secondary Qi channels which connect the Jing to the surface of the body and also to the bone marrow. Jing and Luo are considered to be Qi rivers and streams in the body.

In addition to Jing and Luo, there are eight vessels which serve as balancing channels and are considered to be Qi reservoirs in the body. Some of these vessels also circulate Qi, although their function is different from Jing and Luo. Their function is to regulate the amount of Qi flow in the twelve channels. Among these eight vessels the Ren (Conception Vessel, 任脈) and Du (Governing Vessel, 督脈) are most important. As you remember from earlier chapters, these two vessels play a primary role in Small and Grand Circulation.

Acupuncture theory classifies the internal organs as viscera and bowels. According to this theory, viscera are the organs that store essential substances for the body's use. The viscera are the lungs, kidney, liver, heart, spleen, and pericardium (Baoluo, 包絡). The bowels are organs which do not store substances, but eliminate them, being essentially hollow. The bowels are the large intestine, gall bladder, urinary bladder, small intestine, stomach, and triple burner (Sanjiao, 三焦). Viscera are Yin, and bowels are Yang, and they are grouped in pairs which are closely related to each other. It is important to note that in Chinese medicine, the term "organ" refers more to the functional system of that organ than to the actual physical lump of flesh. Hence, two of the organs in the Chinese system, the pericardium and the triple burner, have no corresponding organ in the Western system.

In classifying Qi channels, there are six degrees of Yin and Yang used to describe the six channels that terminate in the hands and the six that end in the feet. The Yin channels are Taiyin (太陰), Shaoyin (少陰), and Jueyin (厥陰). Taiyin is the very strongest most vigorous Yin. Shaoyin contains some Yang, and Jueyin is exhausted Yin and is found where two Yin channels meet. The Yang channels are Taiyang (太陽), Shaoyang (少陽), and Yangming (陽明). Taiyang is very strong, young Yang. Shaoyang is Yang that has begun to deteriorate, and Yangming is extreme Yang, and is found where two Yang channels meet.

In Yin and Yang theory, Yang is characterized by the outside of things, while Yin is the inside. In consonance with this principle, the twelve channels are considered Yin or Yang depending on whether they are found on the inside or on the outside of the arms or legs. There are three Yin channels on the inside of each arm and leg, and three Yang channels on the outside. Of the two main vessels that make up Small Circulation, the Ren Mai (Conception Vessel, 任脈) is found on the front of the body and is considered Yin. The Du Mai (Governing Vessel, 督脈), is found on the back, and is considered Yang.

Qi circulates within this system of channels and vessels continuously, from the surface to the interior and back to the surface. The paths of the channels are as follows:

Upper Limb—Yin Jing (陰經), movement is from the chest to the hand.

Hand Taiyin Lung (Shou Taiyin Fei Jing, 手太陰肺經). Runs from the top of the chest, along the inside of the arm, and ends on the outside of the thumb.

Hand Shaoyin Heart (Shou Shaoyin Xin Jing, 手少陰心經). Runs from the armpit, down the inside arm, and ends in the little finger.

Hand Jueyin Pericardium (Shou Jueyin Baoluo Jing, 手厥陰包絡經).

Starts in the chest, runs up the chest, then down the middle of the inner arm and ends at the middle finger.

Upper Limb—Yang Jing (陽經), movement is from the hand to the head.

Hand Taiyang Small Intestine (Shou Taiyang Xiao Chang, 手太陽小腸). Starts at the end of the little finger, then runs up the outside of the arm, behind the shoulder, across the neck, and ends in front of the ear.

Hand Shaoyang Triple Burner (Shou Shaoyang San Jiao, 手少陽三焦). Starts at the tip of the ring finger, then runs up the outside of the arm, around the shoulder, over the ear, and ends near the outside of the eyebrow.

Hand Yangming Large Intestine (Shou Yangming Da Chang, 手陽明大腸). Starts at the tip of the index finger, runs along the outside of the arm, and ends near the nose.

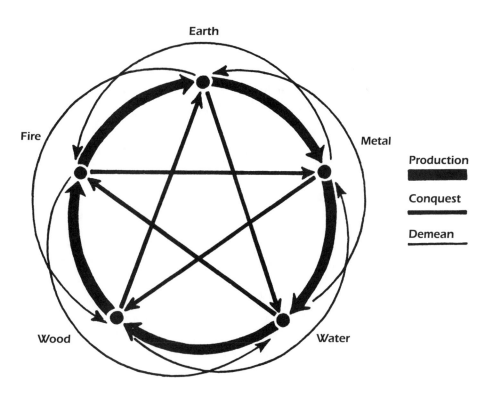

Figure 4-6. Relationships of Five Internal Organs with the Five Elements

Lower Limb—Yin Jing (陰經), movement is from the foot to the chest.

Foot Taiyin Spleen (Zu Taiyin Pi, 足太陰脾). Starts at the tip of the big toe, runs up the inside of the leg, and ends at the top of the chest.

Foot Shaoyin Kidney (Zu Shaoyin Shen, 足少陰腎). Starts under the little toe, rises along the inside of the leg, and ends near the collarbone.

Foot Jueyin Liver (Zu Jueyin Gan, 足厥陰肝). Starts on the outside of the big toe, then the inside of the leg, up the trunk, and ends near the nipple.

Lower Limb—Yang Jing (陽經), movement is from the head to the foot.

Foot Taiyang Bladder (Zu Taiyang Pang Guang, 足太陽膀胱). Starts at the inner corner of the eye, runs over the head, splits and runs in two channels down the back, joins on the back of the thigh and ends on the little toe.

Foot Shaoyang Gall Bladder (Zu Taiyang Dan, 足少陽膽). Starts at the outer corner of the eye, travels over the head, around the back of the shoulder, down the side of the chest and the outside of the leg, and ends in the fourth toe.

Foot Yangming Stomach (Zu Yangming Wei, 足陽明胃). Starts under the eye, runs down the front of the body, then down the outer front of the leg, and ends up in the second toe.

Jing are connected with one another at the extremities, where Yin meets Yang, and at the chest and face, where Yin meets Yin and Yang meets Yang (see Table 4-2). For the purposes of this table, the circuit starts above the nipples, moving through the channels in the order shown. Remember that there are two symmetrical systems, one on each side of the body.

Table 4-2

Order of Qi Circulation

From	To	Channel	Time Period
Top of Chest	Outside of Thumb	Hand Taiyin Lung	3 to 5 AM (Yin, 寅)
Tip of Index Finger	Side of Nose	Hand Yangming Large Intestine	5 to 7 AM (Mao, 卯)
Under the Eye	Second Toe	Foot Yangming Stomach	7 to 9 AM (Chen, 辰)
Big Toe	Top of Chest	Foot Taiyin Spleen	9 to 11 AM (Si, 巳)
Armpit	Little Finger	Hand Shaoyin Heart	11 AM to 1 PM (Wu, 午)
Little Finger	Front of Ear	Hand Taiyang Small Intestine	1 to 3 PM (Wei, 未)
Inner Corner of Eye	Little Toe	Foot Taiyang Bladder	3 to 5 PM (Shen, 申)
Little Toe	Collarbone	Foot Shaoyin Kidney	5 to 7 PM (Qiu, 酉)
Chest	Middle Finger	Hand Jueyin Pericardium	7 to 9 PM (Shu, 戌)
Ring Finger	Outside of Eyebrow	Hand Shaoyang Triple Burner	9 to 11 PM (Hai, 亥)
Outside Corner of the Eye	Fourth Toe	Foot Shaoyang Gall Bladder	11 PM to 1 AM (Zi, 子)
Outside of Big Toe	Side of Nipple	Foot Jueyin Liver	1 to 3 AM (Chou, 丑)

Acupuncture theory also relates the organs to the five elements (Wuxing, 五行): metal (Jin, 金), wood (Mu, 木), water (Shui, 水), fire (Huo, 火), and earth (Tu, 土). These relationships are shown in Table 4-3 and Figure 4-6. The five element theory is used to describe how organ systems influence each other through constructive and destructive sequences.

Table 4-3

Relationship of Internal Organs with the Elements

Five Elements	Metal	Water	Wood	Fire	Earth	Mutual Fire
Yang Channels (External)	Hand Yangming	Foot Taiyang	Foot Shaoyang	Hand Taiyang	Foot Yangming	Hand Shaoyang
Bowels	Large Intestine	Bladder	Gall Bladder	Small Intestine	Stomach	Triple Burner
Yin Channels (Internal)	Hand Taiyin	Foot Shaoyin	Foot Jueyin	Hand Shaoyin	Foot Taiyin	Hand Juyin
Viscera	Lung	Kidney	Liver	Heart	Spleen	Pericardium

From the Qi circulation and its relationship to the environment, the Chinese physicians found that a healthy person should not be too Yin or too Yang. When a person is ill, the acupuncturist will use needling or a few other methods to regulate the Qi flow and bring the person back to health. You should understand that it is not only the cavities lying on the channel corresponding to the afflicted organ that are used. Since the channels are interconnected and affect each other in various ways, cavities throughout the body are used to rebalance particular organs. To do this, an acupuncturist must understand the relation of Qi flow to the seasons and the time of day, as well as the interrelationship of the channels.

In the case of non-organ problems, such as muscle pain or a joint injury, the acupuncturist will usually needle cavities near the injury which are not on the channels (remember, almost half the known cavities are not located on channels). This kind of treatment will increase the Qi circulation in the injured area and remove the stagnant Qi.

This has been only the briefest of introductions to the principles of acupuncture. The author hopes that you are able to gain a basic knowledge of Qi circulation. If you are interested in further research, there are many books available. The following are suggested:

The Theoretical Foundation of Chinese Medicine Systems of Correspondence, by Manfred Porkert, MIT Press, Cambridge, Massachusetts and London, 1978.

Acupuncture—A Comprehensive Text, Shanghai College of Traditional Medicine. Translated and edited by John O'Connor and Dan Bensky, Eastland Press, Chicago, 1981.

4-4. Massage and Rubbing

Massage

People have always instinctively rubbed sore muscles and other painful areas to ease their pain and to help the sore muscle recover more quickly. Long ago it was found that this kind of rubbing can also cure a number of disorders such as headaches, joint pain, and an uneasy stomach, and that simple rubbing can even strengthen weakened organs.

The therapeutic effects of massage are known world-wide. The Japanese have used acupressure, which is derived from Chinese massage, for centuries. The Greek upper classes have used a form of massage—slapping the skin with switches—to cure various disorders. However, the Chinese have fully system-atized massage to agree with the theory of Qi circulation.

There are three general Chinese massage treatments. The first is massaging the muscle; the second, massaging the cavities, or acupuncture points; and the third, massaging the nerve and channel endings. Each category of massage has its own specific uses, but generally a mixture of the three is used.

Muscle massage is used to relieve soreness and bruises. The masseuse fol-lows the direction of the muscle fiber using rubbing, pressing, sliding, grasping, slapping, and shaking techniques. The result is an increase in the circulation of blood and Qi on the skin and in the muscle area. It also helps to spread accu-mulated acid, which collects in the muscles due to hard exercise, or blood (in the case of bruises), or stagnant Qi, allowing the circulation to disperse them more quickly. Commonly this type of massage is also used to help a person overcome a feeling of weakness or tiredness.

The second category is massaging the acupuncture points. These same points are used in Japanese acupressure, with the addition of a few other points. The principle of massaging the acupuncture points is the same as in acupuncture theory: to stimulate the channels by stimulating cavities that can be reached easily by rubbing or pressing with the hands, rather than needles. In acupressure, some non-channel points are used to stimulate minor Qi chan-nels to help circulate energy locally. Figures 4-7 through 4-12 show the common acupuncture points used in massage.

The third category of massage is to rub or press the endings of the nerves and Qi channels. These channels are located on the hands (Figure 4-13), feet (Figure 4-14), and ears (Figure 4-5). You can easily rub the zones that corre-spond to the different organs, or that are effective for specific symptoms or ill-nesses. This form of massage is known in the West as reflexology. Theoretically, if the channel endings are rubbed, the Qi will be stimulated to a higher level, which increases the circulation and benefits the related organ or cures the ill-ness. If you are interested in knowing more about massage, please refer to the book: *Chinese Qigong Massage*, available from YMAA Publication Center.

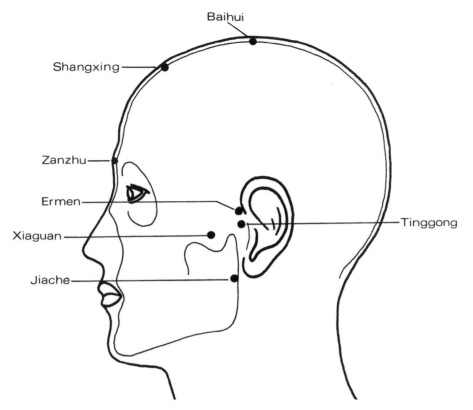

Figure 4-7. Acupuncture Points on the Head Used for Massage

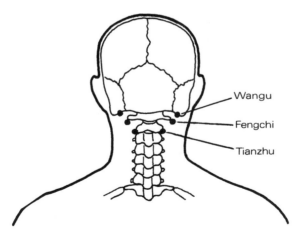

Figure 4-8. Acupuncture Points on the Neck Used for Massage

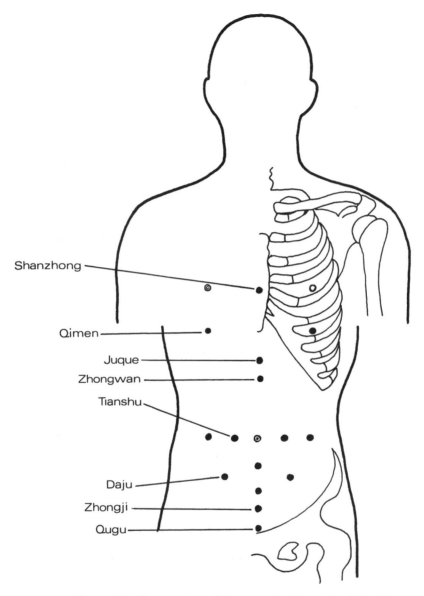

Figure 4-9. Acupuncture Points on the Front Used for Massage

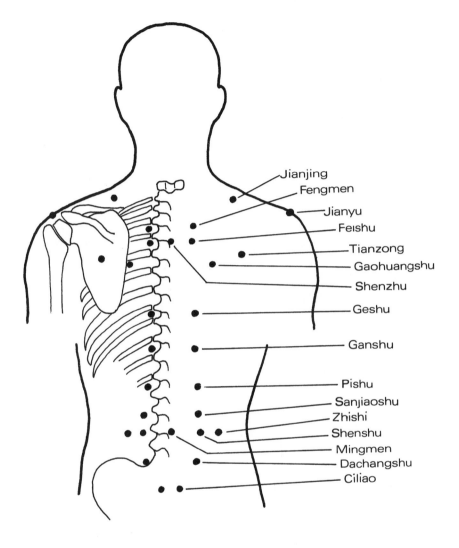

Jianjing
Fengmen
Jianyu
Feishu
Tianzong
Gaohuangshu
Shenzhu
Geshu
Ganshu
Pishu
Sanjiaoshu
Zhishi
Shenshu
Mingmen
Dachangshu
Ciliao

Figure 4-10. Acupuncture Points on the Back Used for Massage

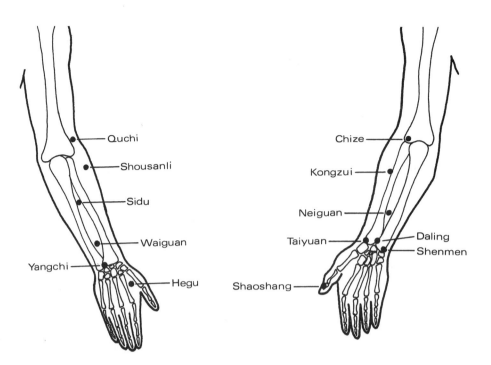

Figure 4-11. Acupuncture Points on the Arms Used for Massage

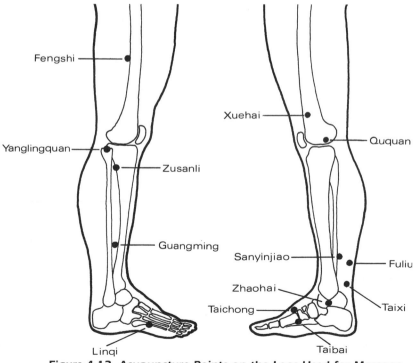

Figure 4-12. Acupuncture Points on the Legs Used for Massage

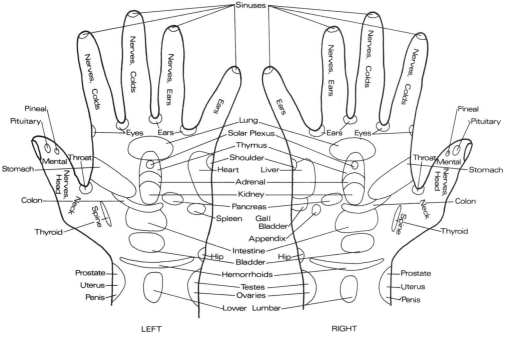

Figure 4-13. Massaging Zones in Hands Reflexology

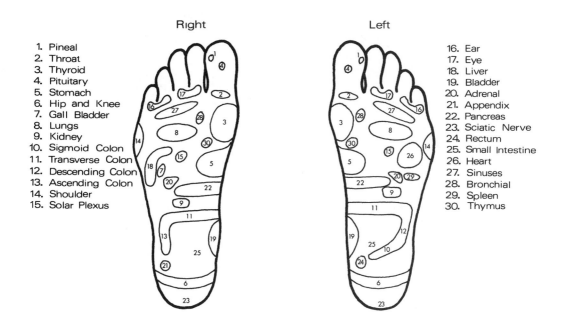

Right   Left

1. Pineal
2. Throat
3. Thyroid
4. Pituitary
5. Stomach
6. Hip and Knee
7. Gall Bladder
8. Lungs
9. Kidney
10. Sigmoid Colon
11. Transverse Colon
12. Descending Colon
13. Ascending Colon
14. Shoulder
15. Solar Plexus

16. Ear
17. Eye
18. Liver
19. Bladder
20. Adrenal
21. Appendix
22. Pancreas
23. Sciatic Nerve
24. Rectum
25. Small Intestine
26. Heart
27. Sinuses
28. Bronchial
29. Spleen
30. Thymus

Figure 4-14. Massaging Zones in Feet Reflexology

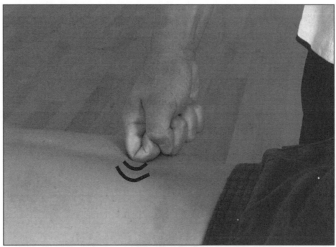

Figure 4-15

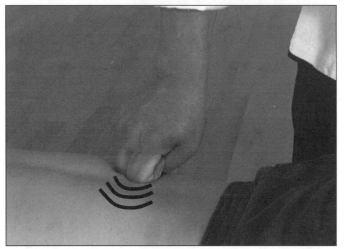

Figure 4-16

Hand Forms and Common Methods Used in Massage.

1. Knuckles: single, double, and four fingers for circular rubbing and pressing (Figures 4-15 to 4-17).
2. The side of the fist for circular rubbing (Figure 4-18).
3. Fingertips for tapping and circular rubbing (Figure 4-19).

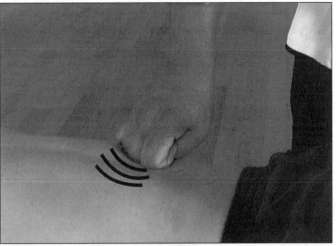

Figure 4-17

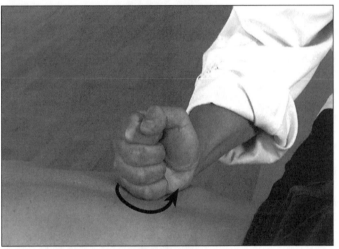

Figure 4-18

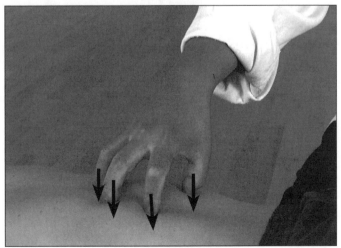

Figure 4-19

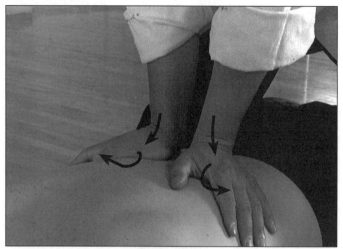

Figure 4-20

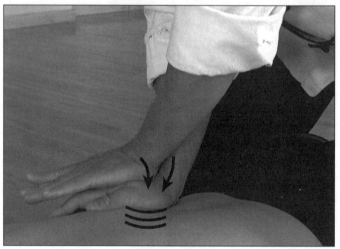

Figure 4-21

Hand Forms and Common Methods Used in Massage—*Continued*

4. The root of the palm (base of the thumb) for circular and straight rubbing and pressing (Figures 4-20 and 4-21).

5. The base of the fingers for circular and straight rubbing and pressing (Figures 4-22 and 4-23).

6. The side of the palm for pressing and rubbing (Figure 4-24).

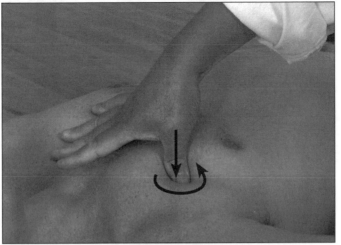

Figure 4-22

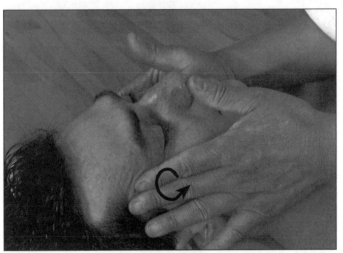

Figure 4-23

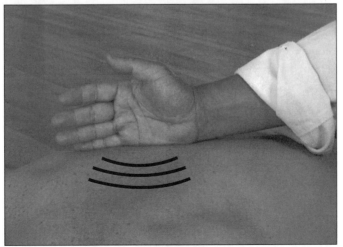

Figure 4-24

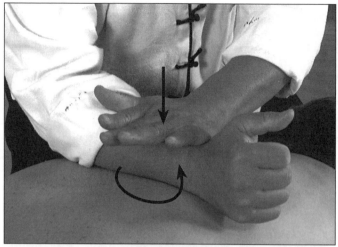

Figure 4-25

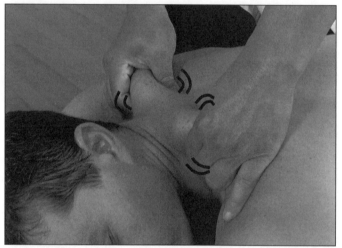

Figure 4-26

Hand Forms and Common Methods Used in Massage—*Continued*

7. The elbow for circular rubbing and pressing (Figure 4-25).

8. Fingers for grasping muscles (Figures 4-26 to 4-28).

9. Pinching or grasping the skin and shaking (Figure 4-29).

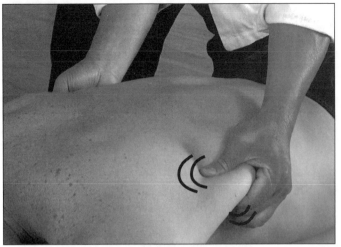

Figure 4-27

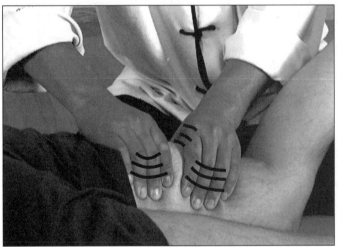

Figure 4-28

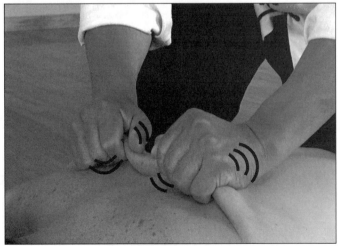

Figure 4-29

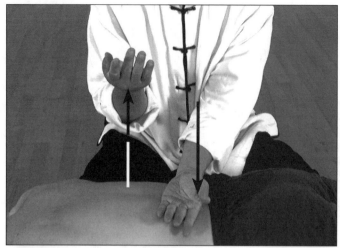

Figure 4-30

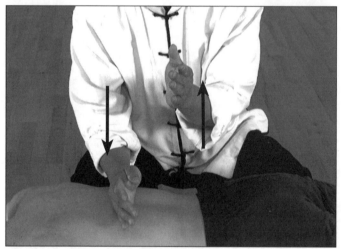

Figure 4-31

Hand Forms and Common Methods Used in Massage—*Continued*

10. Slapping with the backs or the sides of the hands (Figures 4-30 and 4-31).

Rubbing

Very often, when you have an injury such as a bruise or strained joint, you will automatically rub the injured area. This rubbing reduces pain and eases the nerves and muscles. Theoretically, this kind of rubbing causes the Qi to circulate, which in turn prevents Qi stagnation in that area.

In Qigong, rubbing or friction is used to increase heat or Qi on the skin, which increases the energy potential there, and causes Qi to circulate deeper into the body. Rubbing your face correctly can help keep the skin looking youthful by keeping it well nourished with the flow of Qi and blood. As was mentioned earlier, some parts of the body such as the palm (Figure 4-13) and the sole of the foot (Figure 4-14) have channels ending there, and rubbing these channel endings will increase the energy flow in the channels and benefit the corresponding organs. A good example of this is that rubbing the palms together briskly in cold weather will not just keep the arms and hands warm, but the internal organs as well. This is different from massaging the channel zones, which was described in the previous section.

Rubbing the skin over some of the organs will increase the function of the organs through the increased local energy flow caused by the rubbing. For example, rubbing the stomach will lessen pain and increase digestion. Rubbing will also relax the nerves in the area. The same principle holds true for the kidneys.

The large joints of the body—shoulders, elbows, wrists, knees, and ankles—are easily injured by over-exercise or excessive stress on the ligaments. When such injuries do not heal completely, arthritis commonly results. Rubbing the joint area will relax the joint area while stimulating energy circulation, which helps the injured area to heal. In addition, rubbing may even help to cure arthritis after it has set in. For more information on treating arthritis with Qigong, please refer to the book *Arthritis—The Chinese Way of Healing & Prevention*, available from YMAA Publication Center.

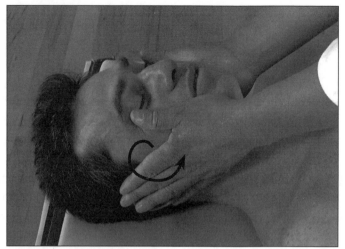

Figure 4-32

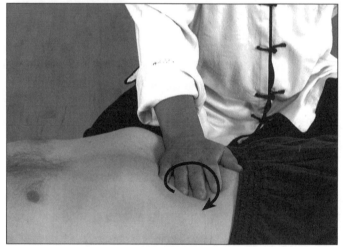

Figure 4-33

Rubbing methods appropriate to each area of the body.

1. Face: Lightly rub the eyelids and eye sockets with the fingertips in a circular motion. Rub the cheeks with light strokes of the fingertips from the nose outward to the sides of the face (Figure 4-32).

2. Stomach: Use a circular motion to harmonize with the curve of the intestines (Figures 4-33 and 4-34).

3. Feet: Rub and press the zones shown in Figure 4-14 (Figure 4-35).

4. Hands: Rub and press the zones shown in Figure 4-13 (Figure 4-36).

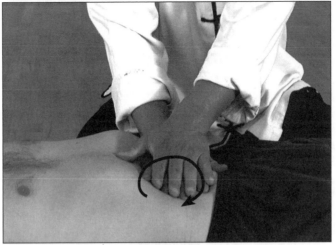

Figure 4-34

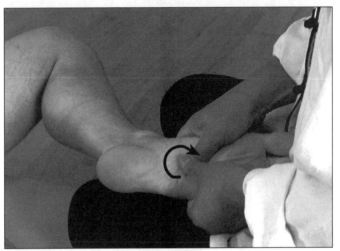

Figure 4-35

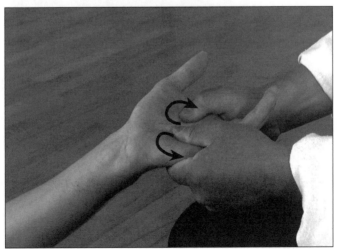

Figure 4-36

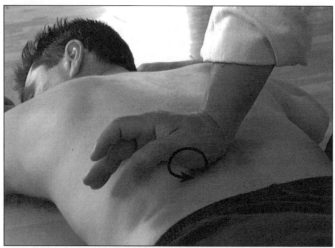

Figure 4-37

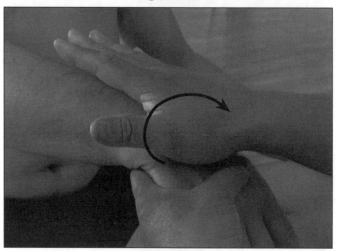

Figure 4-38

Rubbing methods appropriate to each area of the body—*Continued*

5. Kidneys: Rub with a circular motion using the sides of the palm (Figure 4-37).

6. Wrists: For joint rubbing, the main purpose is to warm the joint, not to stimulate the muscles. Rub the wrist by stroking it along the direction of the arm and in a circular motion around the joint (Figure 4-38).

7. Elbows: Rub lightly both up and down the arms and around the arms (Figures 4-39 and 4-40).

8. Shoulders: Rub lightly both up and down the arms and in a circular motion (Figure 4-41).

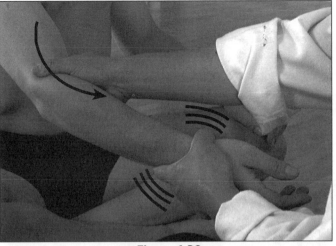

Figure 4-39

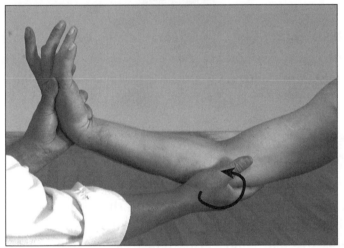

Figure 4-40

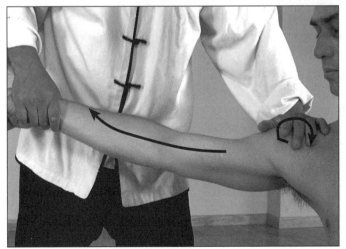

Figure 4-41

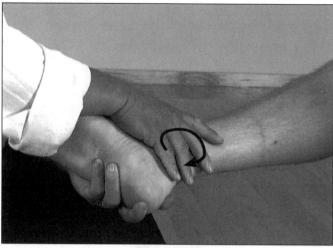

Figure 4-42

Rubbing methods appropriate to each area of the body—*Continued*

9. Knees: Rub lightly both up and down the legs and in a circular motion.

10. Ankles: Rub lightly both up and down the legs and around the joints. Also rub and press the zones shown in Figure 4-14 (Figure 4-42).

4-5. Other Medical Qigong Practices for Good Health

Swinging the Arms (Bai Bi) 擺臂

In the last fifty years an exercise based on the principles of the Yi Jin Jing (易筋經) has become popular. Although the exercise is very simple, the results in strengthening the body and curing illnesses are significant. Theoretically, when you repeatedly swing your arms, the nerves and Qi channels in the shoulder joints are stimulated to a higher state, and this Qi will flow to the areas of lower potential to complete the circulation. Because a number of the Qi channels connected with the different organs terminate in the hands, swinging the arms increases the circulation in these channels. Arm swinging will not only increase the Qi circulation, but the relaxed up and down motion will also increase the flow of blood. This is the same principle of Wai Dan as described in chapter 2.

From the last fifty years of experience, we know that a number of illnesses can be cured simply by frequent practice of swinging the arms. For some cancers, the increase in Qi circulation will help the degenerated cells to function

138

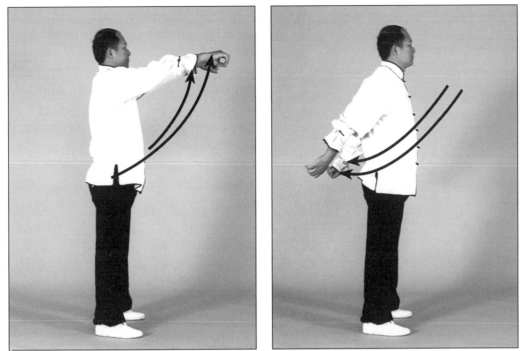

Figure 4-43   Figure 4-44

normally and may help the cancer. According to Qi theory, cancers are caused by the stagnation of Qi and blood, which results in changes to the structure of the cell. Several types of cancer that may be cured by swinging the arms are cancers of the lungs, esophagus, and lymph. Other kinds of disorders that can be helped by swinging the arms are: hardening of the liver, paralysis caused by high blood pressure, high blood pressure itself, heart trouble, and nervous disorders.

The method is very simple. Stand with your feet shoulder width apart, with the tip of your tongue touching the roof of your mouth. Swing your arms forward until they are horizontal with the palms facing down (Figure 4-43), then swing them backwards as far as possible with the palms facing up (Figure 4-44). Keep your entire body relaxed. Start with two hundred to three hundred repetitions, then gradually increase to one or two thousand, or up to half an hour.

Walking in Place

Many Qi channels terminate in the feet and pass through the hip joints. Walking in place has many of the benefits of swinging the arms for similar reasons. As a matter of fact, you can do both at the same time.

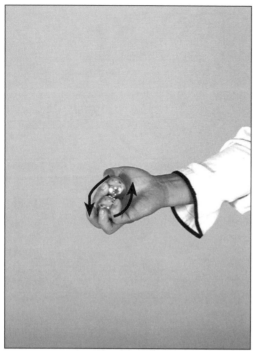

Figure 4-45

Treading Bamboo

Stepping on bamboo rods will stimulate your feet where several channel endings are located. This practice is almost like massage, and the principle is the same. Many health stores sell small wooden rollers that are designed for this purpose. Experiments have even shown that this exercise can help some people grow taller.

Exercise Taiji Balls

In China, you can see people holding two metal Taiji balls, the size of ping pong balls, in one hand and rolling them around. This has the same effect as a hand massage. It stimulates and develops the finger and palm muscles and stimulates the reflexology zones (Figure 4-45) of the palms. The balls are especially good for people who are bedridden and cannot do other exercises.

The Six Sounds

Certain sounds can affect the circulation of Qi. People have always made sounds when ill or distressed. The sounds are the same for all people around the world. Basically, the function of these sounds is to relieve the internal organs of distress through the lungs. Chinese physicians have investigated the matter scientifically, and found that different sounds will affect different organ systems, and high and low tones of a sound will affect the same system differently. Buddhist and Daoist publications describe how different sounds, with varying pitch, are used to relieve or cure several illnesses.

The Daoist documents consulted are: *Tai Shang Yu Zhou Zhen Jing* (太上玉軸真經) by Huang, Ting-Shan (黃庭山), and the *Qian Ji Fang* (千金方) by Sun, Si-Miao (孫思邈) from the Sui and Tang dynasties (589-907 A.D.). The Buddhist texts are the *Xiao Zhi Guan* (小止觀) by a Buddhist named Zhi Zhe Da Shi (智者大師) of Tian Tai Zong (天台宗) and the *Shan Po Luo Mi* (禪波羅密) passed down from Fo Shan (Buddha Mountain, 佛山).

The following table (Table 4-4) lists the six sounds, their corresponding organ, season, element, external body part, and kind of disorder helped. The six sounds should be done in one continuous breath. This will cause a chain relaxation of the corresponding organs. The sounds should not be loud. When a loud sound is made, the corresponding organ will become tight and this will stagnate the Qi circulation. The sounds should be soft, barely audible, and relaxed.

Table 4-4

Sound	He (呵)	Hu (呼)	Si (呬)	Xi (嘻)	Xu (噓)	Chui (吹)
Organ	Heart	Spleen	Lung	Triple Burner	Liver	Kidney
Season	Summer	Four Seasons	Autumn	Internal Fire	Spring	Winter
Element	Fire	Earth	Metal	Mutual Fire	Wood	Water
Body Part	Tongue	Stomach	Skin	Chest	Eyes	Ear
Disorders	Heart Burn Dry mouth Thirst	Indigestion Diarrhea	Cold Cough	Chest Pain	Burning Liver Red Eyes	Waist Pain Joint Pain

Chapter 5
Martial Arts Applications

武學上之應用

5-1. Introduction

The Chinese have studied and developed the martial arts for more than four thousand years. In the beginning, only techniques using brute muscular power were trained. It was not until about 200 B.C., when the circulation of Qi and the use of acupuncture became well understood, that the martial application of Qi began. The attention devoted to it increased significantly when Da Mo's Wai Dan exercises were introduced at the Shaolin Temple in 536 A.D. Although the Yi Jin Jing exercise was intended to be used only for the improvement of health, it was only natural that the monks applied this to the martial arts. Learning martial arts was a necessity of the time in order to protect the temple property and for traveling. The monks found that the Yi Jin Jing training greatly increased the strength and efficiency of their muscles. The training also allowed them to direct Qi to parts of their body to resist blows. From that time on, the use of Wai Dan to develop Qi and to improve the martial arts has been widely researched and developed.

Once it became known that a balanced, unimpeded flow of Qi was necessary for life and well being, the next step of martial Qi training was to find ways to affect an enemy's Qi flow. Martial arts masters found that of the several hundred acupuncture cavities, 108 were easily affected by striking, pressing, grabbing, or kicking, and techniques were developed for this purpose.

Hitting cavities to cause death, unconsciousness or paralysis is called Cavity Strike or Cavity Press (Dian Xue, 點穴). Striking an enemy in such a way as to cause either the windpipe to be obstructed or the lungs or diaphragm to be cramped, so the person cannot breathe, is called Sealing the Breath (Bi Qi, 閉氣). Striking or pressing cavities so that the supply of blood to the brain is obstructed, causing unconsciousness, is called Sealing the Vein (Duan Mai, 斷脈). These techniques are considered the highest art in Chinese Gongfu.

In order to give the martial artist the strength to penetrate to the cavities, the hands and fingers were conditioned and trained by such methods as Iron Sand Palm (Tie Sha Zhang, 鐵砂掌) and Secret Sword (Jian Jue, 劍訣). Training methods to develop penetration power were also created, such as punching at a candle flame and slapping a cloth.

Martial artists who practiced Nei Dan exercises for many years could move energy outside their bodies. Using cavities, they were able to put Qi into a person's system or take it out. This meant they could do cavity strikes without toughening their bodies and without using much force—perhaps with only a touch. This art has fallen into disuse over the centuries, and there are few people today with this ability.

As mentioned above, Qigong was also used by the Shaolin monks to toughen the body to an extent that seems incredible to most Westerners. An adept could withstand strong blows, edged weapons, and even cavity press, but not, of course, bullets. In Gongfu this is called Iron Shirt (Tie Bu Shan, 鐵布衫) or Golden Bell Cover (Jin Zhong Zhao, 金鐘罩).

In this chapter we will briefly discuss cavity press, sealing the vein, sealing the breath, and Iron Shirt or Golden Bell Cover. The Qi cycle and cavity points will also be briefly discussed. If you are interested in more information on cavity location, Qi circulation, and cavity press techniques, refer to the author's book *Shaolin Chin Na*. A detailed description of these techniques requires a separate book to explain the training methods, exact location of cavities, anatomy, theory, attacking methods, etc. The author hopes to publish such a book in the future.

5-2. Cavity Press

The technique of Cavity Press (Dian Xue, 點穴) is probably the highest accomplishment of Qigong in the martial arts. Ever since Qi was understood, martial artists have used various methods to affect an enemy's Qi, either instantly or with a delayed reaction, with the object of causing death, unconsciousness, stupefaction, or numbness of a body area.

In the course of their research, Chinese martial artists have found 108 cavities that can be attacked. There are seventy-two that are considered minor cavities because they cannot be used to kill an opponent, and thirty-six which are vital cavities because it is possible to kill someone by striking one of them at the right time with the correct force.

In striking cavities, the time of day must be right for the strike to be effective, and the exact spot must be struck. Also, the correct hand form must be used. For example, some cavities can be successfully affected by a strike with the knee, while others require a strike with one finger. The force must be sufficient to affect the channel and penetrate to the right depth, because while some cavities are very close to the surface, others are deeper within the body.

Therefore, in order to use cavity strikes effectively, you must first know acupuncture channels, nerves, and anatomy; second, you must know the theory of Qi circulation in relation to the time of day; and third, you must be trained in hand and leg forms and power development. You must also know the techniques for curing cavity press attacks. If the enemy is not dead from an attack, or if a friend has been attacked, there are techniques for reviving them. In many cases, unconscious people can be revived with just a push, pinch, or massage in the correct spot.

Principles of Cavity Press

Cavity Press is a technique in which you affect an opponent's Qi or blood circulation by striking a cavity with a finger, palm, fist, foot, or elbow, or by grasping. When a cavity is correctly struck, several things can happen:

1. The strike can affect Qi circulation and can cause the failure of the corresponding internal organ. For example, a strike to the armpit, affecting the heart channel, will shock the heart, just like a blow to the funny bone affects the arm.

2. The strike can affect both Qi circulation and blood circulation. When the cavity is struck, the muscles around it cramp and cut off blood flow. If the force is sufficient and affects an artery, the artery can rupture, usually resulting in death. For example, a strike to the temple will both shock the brain and possibly rupture the carotid artery. A weak blow to the temple cavity will cause unconsciousness.

3. The strike can directly affect an internal organ. This category of striking is sometimes called Qi Guan Da (器官打) or Organ Striking. For example, a strike to the solar plexus will shock the heart and can cause death. Another example is a strike to the liver, which can cause the muscles around it to cramp and damage the liver. Sufficient force will rupture it. The liver and kidneys are especially susceptible to this kind of attack.

For a number of cavities, a strike will not result in any obvious injury. However, the strike causes the Qi to stagnate in that area, and the person will become ill or die at some later time, perhaps one or two months or even one year in the future. For example, strikes to spinal cavities will generally not show their effect until much later. From anatomy and acupuncture it is known that the spine is the trunk line for the nervous system and the main conduit for Qi. If cavities located in the spinal area are injured, the flow of Qi to the organ related to that part of the spine will be weakened, and eventually organ failure will occur.

There are a number of cavities that can be struck to temporarily disable an enemy. For example, a strike to the Tianzong (天宗) cavity on the shoulder blade will numb both the shoulder and the arm. Another example, known to everyone, is the funny bone, or Shaohai (H-3, 少海) cavity.

The last kind of cavity strike stuns an enemy, causing him to be disoriented or dizzy, or "out on his feet."

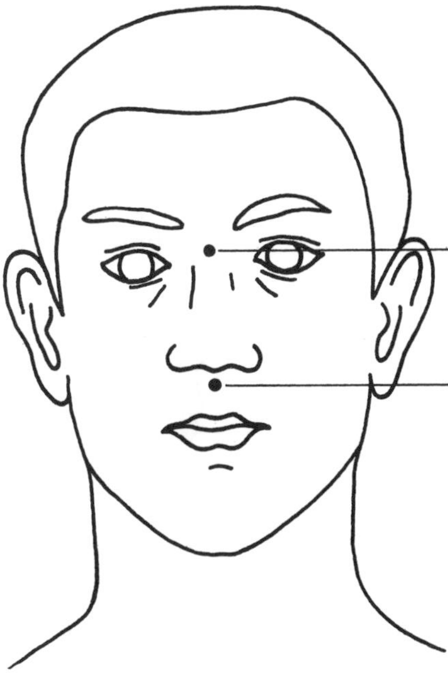

Cavity Press and Time

Because the human body is part of nature, it is affected by the forces at work in the environment. Therefore, the main flow of Qi and blood changes according to the time of day and the season.

Figure 5-1. Cavity Press Cavities on the Face

Generally speaking, during the day the Qi flows most strongly in the front of the body, while at night it flows most strongly in the back. At midnight it is concentrated at the head. Then its focus moves down the front of the body. It is at the solar plexus at noon, and at the perineum at sunset. Then the focus moves up the back and ends at the top of the head again at midnight.

Also, the Qi flow moves from one channel to another every two hours, completing a cycle of the twelve main channels every day. The Governing and Conception vessels are not involved in this cycle. Their flow is constant. Table 5-1 lists the relationship between Qi and blood flow and the time of day.

A martial artist who knows how to coordinate a target with the time of day can easily hurt an opponent in ways that seem mysterious to the uninitiated. Because the martial artist attacks the most intense energies of the body at that particular time, the injury is immediate and drastic.

There are twelve major cavities that are particularly sensitive to attack at specific times. These cavities and their striking times are also listed in Table 5-1, and their locations are illustrated in Figures 5-1 through 5-7. Furthermore, the Qi flow is more predominant in various parts of the body throughout the day. Table 5-1 lists the parts of the body and their times of greatest Qi flow.

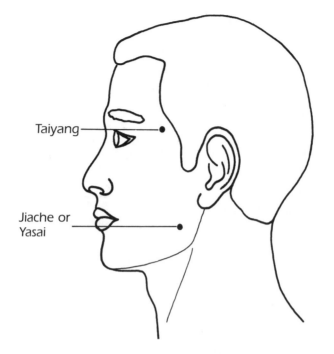

Taiyang

Jiache or
Yasai

Figure 5-2. Cavity Press Cavities on the Side of the Head

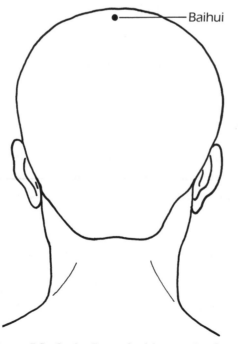

Baihui

Figure 5-3. Cavity Press Cavities on the Crown

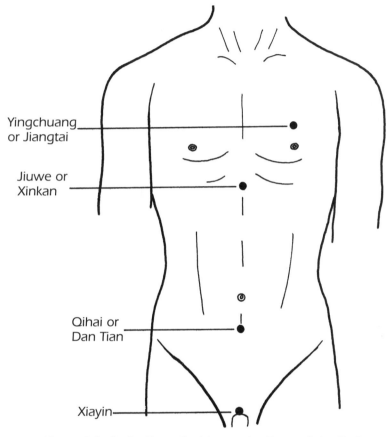

Yingchuang or Jiangtai

Jiuwe or Xinkan

Qihai or Dan Tian

Xiayin

Figure 5-4. Cavity Press Cavities on the Front of the Body

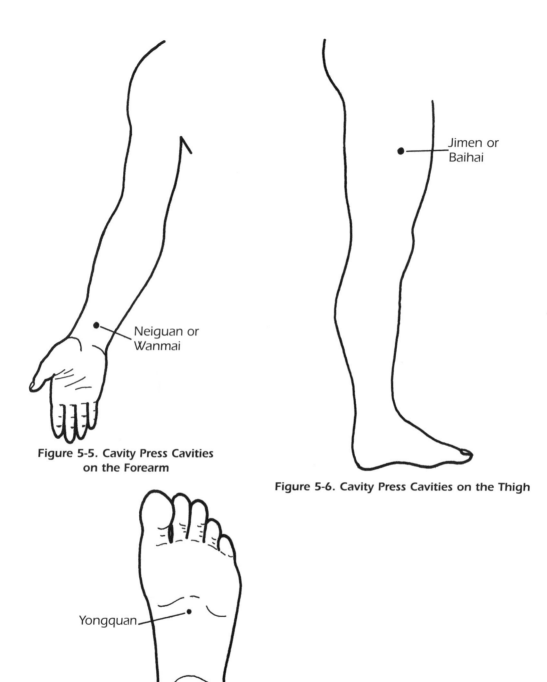

Jimen or
Baihai

Neiguan or
Wanmai

**Figure 5-5. Cavity Press Cavities
on the Forearm**

Figure 5-6. Cavity Press Cavities on the Thigh

Yongquan

**Figure 5-7. Cavity Press Cavities
on the Bottom of the Foot**

Table 5-1

Time	Channel	Body Area	Cavity
11 PM to 1 AM (Zi, 子)	Gall Bladder	Foot	Renzhong (人中)
1 to 3 AM (Chou, 丑)	Liver	Waist	Biliang or Meixin (鼻樑、眉心)
3 to 5 AM (Yin, 寅)	Lung	Eye	Baihui (百會)
5 to 7 AM (Mao, 卯)	Large Intestine	Face	Jiache or Yasai (頰車、牙腮)
7 to 9 AM (Chen, 辰)	Stomach	Head	Taiyang (太陽)
9 to 11 AM (Si, 巳)	Spleen	Hand	Yingchuang or Jiangtai (膺窗、將台)
11 AM to 1 PM (Wu, 午)	Heart	Chest	Neiguan or Wanmai (內關、腕脈)
1 to 3 PM (Wei, 未)	Small Intestine	Stomach	Jiuwei or Xinkan (鳩尾、心坎)
3 to 5 PM (Shen, 申)	Bladder	Heart	Qihai or Dan Tian (氣海、丹田)
5 to 7 PM (Qiu, 酉)	Kidney	Back (Spleen)	Jimen or Baihai (箕門、白海)
7 to 9 PM (Shu, 戌)	Pericardium	Neck (Head)	Xiayin (下陰)
9 to 11 PM (Hai, 亥)	Triple Burner	Leg (Ankle)	Yongquan (湧拳)

5-3. Sealing the Vein and Sealing the Breath

Sealing the Vein (Duan Mai, 斷脈)

Strictly speaking, sealing the vein can also be classified as a cavity press because the vein is sealed by striking a cavity. However, Chinese martial artists consider it separately from cavity press because the injury principle is different. The objective of sealing the vein is to cause unconsciousness or even death by stopping the flow of blood to the head, cutting off the oxygen supply to the brain. Therefore, the cavities used for sealing the vein are mainly located in the neck.

There are two principal ways to seal the vein: striking and compressing. When certain cavities on the neck near the carotid artery are struck, it will affect the Qi circulation in that area and shock the nerves around the cavity. This will in turn cause the muscle to spasm, blocking the artery and completely or partially sealing the blood supply to the brain. When a person does not receive oxygen to the brain for five to ten seconds, he or she will lose consciousness. Another way of sealing the vein is to compress the side of the neck by choking to seal the artery and stop the oxygen supply.

The person whose vein has been sealed can be revived within a few minutes without damage to the brain. Usually, a palm strike to a certain spot on the spine will release the muscle tension in the neck and allow the blood to flow freely again. After the person is revived, a soft massage of the neck muscles will expedite recovery.

Sealing the Breath (Bi Qi, 閉氣)

Sealing the breath is a technique that causes a person to lose consciousness by restricting the supply of air to the lungs so that the person cannot breathe. There are two main categories of sealing the breath. In one, the wind pipe is sealed by being grasped and compressed, which completely stops the lungs from taking in air, thus causing unconsciousness or even death. In the other, the channels around the lungs or the channels which are associated with the lungs are struck. The lungs are protected by the ribs, which are covered with layers of muscles inside and outside. In an ordinary strike, only the muscles on the outside of the ribs are affected. However, if the appropriate cavity on the chest or back is struck, the muscles inside the ribs will also be shocked. They will tighten up and prevent the lungs from expanding and taking in air.

Usually, this type of sealing the breath will cause only a partial sealing of the lungs. Most of the time the person will lose consciousness because of lack of oxygen, but will not die. If an injured person is not revived for a long time, death might result. But generally the person will recover. To speed recovery, apply pressure with the palm to the side of the chest that is not in spasm. This will balance the pressure and help to release the spasm. The person can also be revived by throwing water on him or her.

Sealing the breath can be caused by striking the cavities just above and below the nipple, the solar plexus, the stomach muscles, or any of several cavities on the back.

5-4. Golden Bell Cover or Iron Shirt

Chinese martial artists often demonstrate their ability by bending an iron bar pressed into their throats. They do this by concentrating Qi at the spot the bar is pressing. This is a spectacular way of demonstrating the results of a martial Qigong training system called Iron Shirt (Tie Bu Shan, 鐵布衫) or Golden Bell Cover (Jin Zhong Zhao, 金鐘罩). The reason for these names is that the training will enable a person to resist a blow or punch without injury or pain, as though he or she were wearing an iron shirt or were protected by a golden bell.

This training may have started in the sixth century when Da Mo's Yi Jin Jing (易筋經) began to be used. One of the purposes of Yi Jin Jing training is to concentrate the Qi in a specific area, which will not only increase the muscle power, which is supported by Qi, but will also increase the ability to resist blows, reducing injury to a minimum. This kind of training has continued to be researched and practiced to the present. Because the training of the body's resistance comes from repeated beating, it is also called Beating Endurance (Ai Da, 挨打) training. Another name for this training is Bunch Beating (Pai Da, 排打) because the first few stages of training use bunches of bamboo, wood, and iron wire to hit the body.

The training principle is very simple. You may have noticed that tightening the appropriate muscles in an area where you are about to get hit reduces the pain and injury of the blow. This is the beginning of Iron Shirt training. The reason for this phenomenon is that when muscles are tight, the Qi flow is slow, so the nerve sensation is slow and dull. This stops the pain message from passing to the brain. Additionally, when the muscles are tensed, most of the power of a blow or punch will be stopped by the tensed muscle, so the main Qi channels under the muscles won't be disturbed. Consequently, the injury will be confined to the muscle itself, not to the organs related to the Qi channel.

In order to prevent injury in Iron Shirt training, the practitioner must be conditioned gradually, first the skin and then the muscles. Then, in advanced Iron Shirt, the Qi must be trained to concentrate in the area being struck to repulse the impact. With the Qi supporting the muscle, the Qi channel won't be injured, and so the body can eventually resist even a cavity press.

In order to complete the advanced training, the Wai Dan Qigong training from chapter 2 is extremely important. Also, in order to keep the Qi circulation smooth and complete, Nei Dan should be practiced. Without Wai Dan and Nei Dan training the Iron Shirt will only be on the surface of the body. The body can still be injured when attacked by penetrating power.

There is a martial proverb: "Train the muscles and skin externally, and train Qi internally."[1] This implies that Qigong is the foundation of the training. Qi training can make the internal organs strong and healthy. When Qi is concentrated by the mind, it can be expanded to the entire body (see chapter 3) or focused in a small area to rebound a blow.

In Iron Shirt training, the first step is to beat the skin with minor power with bamboo or rattan strips about one and a half feet long, bound at one end. This striking will stimulate the skin and surface muscles. Because no deep injury can occur, the entire body can be trained in this way. However, for the very beginner, only areas that have a thick layer of muscle to support the blows—the shoulders, stomach, chest, back, thighs, arms, and calves—should be struck. With each strike, the muscle being struck should be tightened and the mind should be concentrated at that spot. This will train Qi concentration and the natural resistant reaction. Only after the above areas can take a strike without feeling pain can other areas such as the shins, knees, head, elbows, etc., be trained. This training should continue until you do not feel pain.

This skin and shallow muscle stimulation will let the nerve system get acclimated to being struck. If a ticklish person were tickled constantly, eventually his nerve system would no longer feel ticklish. This training works the same way.

The next step is to use striking power which can penetrate deeper into the body. For this training, a bunch of iron wire bound at one end is used. Follow the same routine with Qi concentration and muscle tension until the deep muscles can resist the external blows. For this step, since the blow will be stronger and more penetrating, you must have strong Qi to avoid disturbing the Qi flow. Also, herbs should be used to cure the bruises, so that Qi will not become stagnant anywhere.

It is important to note here that all these training methods should be done only with a qualified master who knows how to control the penetration power of the blows, and who also knows how to treat injuries.

Only after the less dangerous areas have been trained, and you have gained enough skill with Qi transport, can other vital areas such as the head, throat, kidneys and liver be trained. Also at this point, the master will stimulate the vital cavities such as the temples, throat, armpits, solar plexus, etc. to train you to protect these areas. Later, these vital cavities will be struck at their most vulnerable times of day. When you can resist a cavity press to a vital area without pain and injury, then you have completed the training.

There are two vital places—the eyes and the groin—where Qi cannot be directed. Therefore, they remain vulnerable even for one who has completed the above training. However, there are some practitioners who are able to pull their testicles up into the abdomen, leaving only their eyes vulnerable.

Reference

1. 外練筋骨皮，內練一口氣。

Conclusion

結 語

The author hopes that this book will help to set you on the right path of Qigong research and development, and will dispel some of the mystery and confusion which still shroud this art.

This book can be only a beginning. It is now up to you to practice and research for yourself.

The information in this book will enable you to lay a good foundation in energy development. Space has limited the presentation of the martial applications of Qigong, but the author hopes to publish more information on this matter in the future. You are also encouraged to seek out qualified masters from which to learn. The author hopes that he has provided a useful overview of this ancient and useful Chinese art.

Appendix A
Translation and Glossary of Chinese Terms

Ai Da 挨打
Means "Beating Endurance." An external iron shirt training method.

Ba Duan Jin 八段錦
Eight Pieces of Brocade. A Wai Dan Qigong practice said to have been created by Marshal Yue Fei during the Southern Song dynasty (1127-1279 A.D.).

Ba Fa 八法
The eight methods of the internal martial style Liu He Ba Fa.

Bai Bi 擺臂
Swinging Arms. A simple Qigong exercise popularly practiced in China.

Bai He 白鶴
Means "White Crane." A southern Chinese martial arts style.

Bao Pu Zi 抱朴子
A well known Qigong and Chinese medical book written by Ge Hong during the Jin dynasty in the 3rd century A.D.

Bao Shen Mi Yao 保身祕要
A Qigong and medical book that describes moving and stationary Qigong practices. It was written by Cao, Yuan-Bai during the Qing dynasty (1644-1911 A.D.).

Bagua (Ba Kua) 八卦
Literally, "Eight Divinations." Also called the Eight Trigrams. In Chinese philosophy, the eight basic variations; shown in the *Yi Jing* as groups of single and broken lines.

Baihui (Gv-20) 百會
Literally, "Hundred Meetings." An important acupuncture cavity located on the top of the head. The Baihui cavity is on the Governing Vessel.

Baoluo 包絡
Pericardium. One of the twelve primary Qi channels in Chinese medicine.

Beng 弸
Expand.

Bi Gang 閉肛
Close the anus.

Bi Qi 閉氣
Seal the breath. A Qin Na technique used to prevent an opponent from taking air into the lungs.

Bi 鼻
Nose.

Bian Que 扁鵲
A well known physician who wrote the book, *Nan Jing (Classic on Disorders)* sometime between the Qin and Han dynasties (221 B.C.-220 A.D.).

Bian Shi 砭石

Stone probes. Used to press acupuncture cavities for healing before metal needles were available.

Biliang 鼻樑

Nose bridge. The upper section of the nose between the eyes.

Chadili 剎帝利

The last name of Da Mo, also known as Bodhidarma.

Cao, Yuan-Bai 曹元白

A well known physician and Qigong master who wrote a book called *Bao Shen Mi Yao (The Secret Important Document of Body Protection)* during the Qing dynasty (1644-1911 A.D.). It describes moving and stationary Qigong practices.

Chan (Zen) 禪，忍

A Chinese school of Mahayana Buddhism which asserts that enlightenment can be attained through meditation, self-contemplation and intuition, rather than through study of scripture. Chan is called Zen in Japan.

Changquan (Chang Chuan) 長拳

Means "Long Range Fist." Changquan includes all northern Chinese long range martial styles. Changquan has also been used to refer to Taijiquan.

Chao, Yuan-Fang 巢元方

A well known physician and Qigong master who lived between the Sui and Tang dynasties (581-907 A.D.). Chao, Yuan-Fang compiled the *Zhu Bing Yuan Hou Lun (Thesis on the Origins and Symptoms of Various Diseases),* which is a veritable encyclopedia of Qigong methods, listing 260 different ways of increasing the Qi flow.

Chen Bo 陳博

The reputed creator of the internal martial art Liu He Ba Fa, during the Song dynasty (960-1280 A.D.) on Hua Shan (Mt. Hua).

Chen, Chang-Xing 陳長興

The fourteenth generation master of Chen Style Taijiquan, who taught the art to Yang, Lu-Shan.

Chen, Ji-Ru 陳繼儒

A well known physician and Qigong master who wrote the book, *Yang Shen Fu Yu (Brief Introduction to Nourishing the Body)* during the Qing dynasty (1644-1911 A.D.). The book describes the three treasures: Jing (essence), Qi (internal energy), and Shen (spirit).

Cheng, Gin-Gsao 曾金灶

Dr. Yang, Jwing-Ming's White Crane master.

Chong Qi 充氣

To fill the Qi.

Chui 丑

To blow.

Chun Qiu Zhan Guo 春秋戰國

Spring and Autumn and Warring States periods (722-222 B.C.).

Da Mo 達摩

The Indian Buddhist monk who is credited with creating the Yi Jin Jing and Xi Sui Jing while at the Shaolin monastery. His last name was Chadili and he was also known as Bodhidarma. He was once the prince of a small tribe in southern India.

Da Mo Wai Dan 達磨外丹

The Wai Dan (External Elixir) Qigong created by Da Mo.

Da Qiao 搭橋
Building the Bridge. It means to touch your tongue on the roof of the mouth.

Da Sheng 大乘
Mahayana, the Great Vehicle, which includes Tibetan Buddhism and Chan or Zen Buddhism, which is very well known to the West.

Da Zhou Tian 大周天
Literally, "Grand Cycle Heaven." Usually called Grand Circulation. After a Nei Dan Qigong practitioner completes Small Circulation, he or she will circulate Qi throughout the entire body or exchange Qi with nature.

Dan Tian 丹田
Literally, "Field of Elixir." Locations in the body which are able to store and generate Qi (elixir) in the body. The Upper, Middle, and Lower Dan Tian are located respectively between the eyebrows, at the solar plexus, and a few inches below the navel.

Dao 道
The "Way," by implication the "Natural Way."

Dao De Jing 道德經
Morality Classic. Written by Lao Zi.

Di Li 地理
Geomancy.

Di Li Shi 地理師
Di Li means "Geomancy" and Shi means "Teacher." Therefore Di Li Shi is a teacher or master who analyzes geographic locations according to the formulas in the *Yi Jing (Book of Changes)* and the energy distributions in the earth. Also called Feng Shui Shi.

Dian Xue 點穴
Dian means "To point and exert pressure" and Xue means "Cavities." Dian Xue refers to those Qin Na techniques which specialize in attacking acupuncture cavities to immobilize or kill an opponent.

Dian Xue massage 點穴按摩
A Chinese massage technique in which the acupuncture cavities are stimulated through pressing. Dian Xue massage is also called acupressure and is the root of Japanese Shiatsu.

Dong Chu 動觸
Literally "Moving Touch." Refers to the unusual, automatic movements or sensations sometimes experienced during Qigong practice. Also called Chu Gan.

Dong, Hai-Chuan 董海川
A well known Chinese internal martial artist who is credited with the creation of Baguazhang in the late Qing dynasty (1644-1911 A.D.).

Du Mai 督脈
Usually translated "Governing Vessel." One of the eight extraordinary vessels.

Duan Mai 斷脈
Duan means "To break" and Mai means "Blood vessel." Duan Mai means to seal or to break the blood vessel.

Duqi 肚臍
The navel.

Emei 峨嵋
A mountain in Sichuan Province, China.

Fan Hu Xi 反呼吸
Reverse Breathing. Also commonly called "Daoist Breathing."

Fan Tong Hu Xi 返童呼吸
Back to Childhood Breathing. Breath training in Nei Dan Qigong through which the practitioner tries to regain control of the muscles in the lower abdomen. Also called "Abdominal Breathing."

Fo Shan 佛山
Buddha mountain. A mountain in Canton Province, China.

Fu Xi 膚息
Skin Breathing.

Ge Hong 葛洪
A famous physician and Qigong master who wrote the book, *Bao Pu Zi* during the Jin dynasty in the 3rd century A.D.

Ge Zhi Yu Lun 格致餘論
The Chinese name of the book *A Further Thesis of Complete Study*. This book is a medical and Qigong thesis written by Zhu, Dan-Xi at some time during the Chinese Song, Jin, and Yuan dynasties (960-1368 A.D.).

Gong (Kung) 功
Energy or hard work.

Gong Shou 拱手
Arc Hands. Also known as "Universal Post." It is a standing meditation form of Qigong training, in which Qi is built up in the shoulders and then circulated to the limbs and internal organs.

Guang Xiao Temple 光孝寺
A temple located in Canton Province, China.

Gongfu (Kung Fu) 功夫
Means "Energy-Time." Anything that takes time and energy to learn or to accomplish is called Gongfu.

Ha 哈
The sound that helps to relieve fevers.

Haidi 海底
Bottom of the Sea. The place between the scrotum or vagina and the anus.

Han Shu Yi Wen Zhi 漢書藝文志
Han's Book of Arts and Scholarship. A book written during the Qin and Han dynasties (255 B.C. to 220 A.D.).

Han dynasty 漢朝
A dynasty in Chinese history (206 B.C.-221 A.D.).

Han, Ching-Tang 韓慶堂
A Chinese martial artist, especially well known in Taiwan in the last forty years. Master Han is also Dr. Yang, Jwing-Ming's Long Fist grand master.

He 呵
One of the six healing sounds. He is used to regulate the Qi imbalance of the heart.

Hebei 河北
A province in China.

Hei 嘿
The sound used to increase a person's working strength.

Henan Province 河南省
The province in China where the Shaolin temple is located.

Hu 呼
One of the six healing sounds. Hu is used to regulate the imbalance of Qi in spleen.

Hu Bu Gong 虎步功
Tiger Step Gong. A style of Qigong training.

Hua Shan 華山
Hua mountain. Located in Hua Yin county, Shanxi Province.

Hua Tuo 華陀
A well known physician from the Chinese Jin dynasty in the 3rd century A.D.

Huan 還
To return.

Huang Di 黃帝
The Yellow Emperor (2690-2590 B.C.).

Huang, Ting-Shan 黃庭山
A Daoist who wrote the book *Tai Shang Yu Zhou Zhen Jing*.

Hubei Province 湖北省
A province in China.

Huiyin (Co-1) 會陰
An acupuncture cavity belonging to the Conception Vessel.

Huo 火
Fire.

Huo Long Gong 火龍功
Fire Dragon Gong. A style of Qigong training created by Taiyang martial stylists.

Huo Lu 火爐
The Furnace. In Daoist Qigong practice it means the Dan Tian.

Ji, Long-Feng 姬隆豐
A martial artist who claimed to have obtained a book, *Quan Jing* or *Fist Fighting Classic*, written by Yue Fei when he visited a hermit on Zhong Nan Mountain at the end of the Ming dynasty (1644 A.D.).

Jiaji 夾脊
Literally, "Squeezing Spine." A location on the upper spine. This place is called Lingtai in acupuncture.

Jian Jue 劍訣
Literally, "Secret Sword." A special hand form for Qigong or sword practice.

Jiangtai 將台
A cavity on the upper back area. Jiangtai is the name used in Chinese martial arts. It is called Yingchuang (S-16) in acupuncture.

Jiao Hua Gong 叫化功
Beggar Gong. A style of Qigong training.

Jin Dan 金丹
Literally, "Golden-Elixir." It means the Qi in the body.

Jin 金
Metal. One of the five elements in Chinese medicine.

Jin 金
A dynasty in China (1115-1134 A.D.).

Jin dynasty 晉
A Chinese dynasty in the third century A.D.

Jin Kui Yao Lue 金匱要略
A Chinese book called *Prescriptions from the Golden Chamber*, which discusses the use of breathing and acupuncture to maintain good Qi flow. This book was written by Zhang, Zhong-Jing between the Qin and Han dynasties (221 B.C.-220 A.D.).

Jin Zhong Zhao 金鐘罩
Literally, "Golden Bell Cover." A higher level of Iron Shirt training.

Jin, Shao-Feng 金紹峰
Dr. Yang, Jwing-Ming's White Crane grand master.

Jing 經
Channels. Sometimes translated as "Meridians." Refers to the twelve organ-related "rivers" in which Qi circulates throughout the body.

Jing Luo Lun 經絡論
Theory of Qi Channels and Branches.

Jiuwei (Co-15) 鳩尾
An acupuncture point in Chinese medicine which belongs to the Conception Vessel. This location is called Xinkan in Chinese marital arts.

Jueyin 厥陰
Exhausted Yin.

Jun Qing 君倩
A Daoist and Chinese doctor from the Jin dynasty (265-420 A.D.). Jun Qing is credited as the creator of the Five Animal Sports Qigong practice.

Kao Tao 高濤
Dr. Yang, Jwing-Ming's first Taijiquan master.

Kou Chi 扣齒
Knocking the teeth. A Qigong practice from the Eight Pieces of Brocade.

Kuo Qi 闊氣
Expanding Qi. The technique of skin breathing.

Lan Shi Mi Cang 蘭室祕藏
Secret Library of the Orchid Room. A Chinese medical and Qigong book written by Li Guo at some time during the Song, Jin, and Yuan dynasties (960-1368 A.D.).

Lao Zi 老子
The creator of Daoism, also called Li Er.

Laogong (P-8) 勞宮
The name of a cavity on the Pericardium Channel in the center of the palm.

Le 勒
Reserve. One of the eight methods in Liu He Ba Fa.

Li Bai 李白
One of the most famous poets in China (701-762 A.D.) who lived during the Tang dynasty (618-907 A.D.).

Li Er 李耳
The nickname of Lao Zi. The creator of scholarly Daoism.

Li Guo 李果
A well known Chinese physician and Qigong master who wrote the book, *Lan Shi Mi Cang (Secret Library of the Orchid Room)* some time during Song, Jin, and Yuan dynasties (960-1368 A.D.).

Li, Mao-Ching 李茂清
Dr. Yang, Jwing-Ming's Long Fist master.

Li, Shi-Zhen 李時珍
Author of the book *The Verifications of the Strange Channels and the Eight Vessels,* which discusses the relationship of Qigong with the channels.

Lian Qi 練氣
Lian means "To train, to strengthen and to refine." It is a Daoist training process through which the Qi grows stronger and more abundant.

Liang dynasty 梁
A dynasty in Chinese history (502-557 A.D.)

Liang Wu emperor 梁武帝
Emperor of the Liang dynasty.

Lingtai (Gv-10) 靈台
An acupuncture cavity belonging to the Governing Vessel.

Liu He 六合
The six combinations or harmonizations of Liu He Ba Fa.

Liu He Ba Fa 六合八法
Literally, "Six Combinations Eight Methods." A Chinese internal martial art, its techniques are combined from Taijiquan, Xingyi and Baguazhang. This internal martial art was reportedly created by Chen Bo during the Song dynasty (960-1279 A.D.).

Long Quan 龍泉
Dragon Spring.

Lu You 陸游
A poet of the Southern Song dynasty (1127-1280 A.D.).

Luo 絡
The small Qi channels which branch out from the primary Qi channels and are connected to the skin and to the bone marrow.

Mai 脈
Means "Vessel" or "Qi Channel."

Meixin 眉心
Literally, "Eyebrow Center." The place between the eyebrows.

Mian 綿
Soft.

Mian Quan 綿拳
Literally, "Soft Fist." Another name for Taijiquan.

Ming dynasty 明朝
A Chinese dynasty from1368 to 1644 A.D.

Ming Tian Gu 鳴天鼓
Beating the heaven drum. A Qigong practice from the Eight Pieces of Brocade.

Mu 木
Wood. One of the five elements.

Nan Hua Jing 南華經
A book written by the Daoist philosopher Zhuang Zi around 300 B.C. This book describes the relationship between health and breathing.

Nan Jing 難經
Classic on Disorders. A medical book written by the famous physician Bian Que between the Qin and Han dynasties (221 B.C.-220 A.D.). *Nan Jing* describes methods of using the breathing to increase Qi circulation.

Naohu (Gv-17) 腦戶
Brain's household. One of the acupuncture cavities belonging to the Governing Vessel.

Nei Dan 內丹
Literally, "Internal Elixir." A form of Qigong in which Qi (the elixir) is built up in the body and spread out to the limbs.

Nei Gong 內功
Means "Internal Gongfu" which implies Qigong practice.

Nei Gong Tu Shuo 內功圖説
Illustrated Explanation of Nei Gong. A Qigong book written by Wang, Zu-Yuan during the Qing dynasty. This book presents the Twelve Pieces of Brocade and explains the idea of combining both moving and stationary Qigong.

Neiguan (P-6) 內關
An acupuncture cavity belonging to the Pericardium primary Qi channel.

Nei Jing 內經
Inner Classic. A Chinese medical book written during the reign of the Yellow Emperor (2690-2590 B.C.).

Nei Shi Gongfu 內視功夫
Nei Shi means "To look internally," so Nei Shi Gongfu refers to the art of looking inside yourself to read the state of your health and the condition of your Qi.

Northern Wei 北魏
One of China's dynasties (386-420 A.D.).

Pai Da 排打
Bunch Beating. A training method from Iron Shirt that uses a bamboo bunch to strike the skin.

Qi (Chi) 氣
The general definition of Qi is: universal energy, including heat, light, and electromagnetic energy. A narrower definition of Qi refers to the energy circulating in human or animal bodies. A current popular model is that the Qi circulating in the human body is bioelectric in nature.

Qi Guan Da 器官打
Organ Striking. A category of attack in Chinese martial arts that aims directly for the internal organs.

Qi Hua Lun 氣化論
Qi Variation Thesis. An ancient treatise which discusses the variations of Qi in the universe.

Qi Huo 起火
To start the fire. In Qigong practice, when you start to build up Qi at the Lower Dan Tian.

Qi Jing Ba Mai 奇經八脈
Literally, "Strange (Odd) Channels Eight Vessels." Usually referred to as the eight extraordinary vessels or simply as the vessels. Called odd or strange because they are not well understood and some of them do not exist in pairs.

Qi Jing Ba Mai Kao 奇經八脈考
Deep Study of the Extraordinary Eight Vessels, written by Li, Shi-Zhen.

Qian Jin Fang 千金方
Thousand Gold Prescriptions. A book written by Sun, Si-Miao that describes a method of guiding Qi, introduces the use of the six sounds and their relationship with the internal organs, and also introduces a collection of massage techniques called Lao Zi's Forty-nine Massage Techniques.

Qie Zhen 切診
Palpation. One of the diagnostic techniques used in Chinese medicine.

Qigong (Chi Kung) 氣功
Gong means "Gongfu" (literally "Energy-Time"). Therefore, Qigong means study, research, and/or practices related to Qi.

Qihai (Co-6) 氣海
An acupuncture cavity belonging to the Conception Vessel.

Qin dynasty 秦朝
A Chinese dynasty from 255-206 B.C.

Qin Na (Chin Na) 擒拿
Literally means "Grab Control." A component of Chinese martial arts that emphasizes grabbing techniques to control an opponent's joints, in conjunction with attacking certain acupuncture cavities.

Qing dynasty 清朝
The last Chinese dynasty (1644-1912 A.D.).

Quan Jing 拳經
Means "Fist Classic."

Ren (Zen) 忍
Means "To endure." The Japanese name of Chan.

Ren Mai 任脈
Conception Vessel. One of the Eight Extraordinary Vessels.

Ren Shi 人事
Literally, "Human Relations." Refers to human events, activities and relationships.

Ren Zong 仁宗
A Song emperor who ruled from 1023-1064 A.D.

Renzhong (Gv-26) 人中
An acupuncture cavity belonging to the Governing Vessel.

Ru Men Shi Shi 儒門視事
The Confucian Point of View. A book written by Zhang, Zi-He during the Song, Jin, and Yuan dynasties (960-1368 A.D.).

San Gong 散功
Literally, "Energy Dispersion." A state of premature degeneration of the muscles where the Qi cannot effectively energize them. It can be caused by over-training.

San Guan 三關
Three Gates. The three key gates through which the Qi must pass in Small Circulation meditation.

San Sheng 三乘
The three conveyances of Buddhism.

Sanjiao 三焦
Triple Burner. One of the twelve organs in Chinese medicine.

Shan Po Luo Mi 禪波羅密
A classic Buddhist text.

Shang Ceng Qi 上層氣
Upper Level Breathing. It means breathing through the lungs.

Shang dynasty 商朝
A dynasty in Chinese history from 1766-1154 B.C.

Shangbei 上背
The upper back.

Shanxi Province 山西省
A province in China.

Shao Shi 少室
A peak of Song Mountain, located in Deng Feng Xian of Henan Province.

Shaohai (H-3) 少海
An acupuncture cavity belonging to heart primary Qi channel.

Shaolin 少林
Literally "Young Woods." The name of the Shaolin Temple.

Shaolin Temple 少林寺
A monastery located in Henan Province, China. The Shaolin Temple is well known because of its martial arts training.

Shaolin Wu Xing Quan 少林五形拳
Shaolin Five Animal Fists. These five animals include the tiger, the leopard, the dragon, the snake, and the crane.

Shaoyang 少陽
Lesser Yang.

Shaoyin 少陰
Lesser Yin.

Shen 神
Spirit. According to Chinese Qigong, the Shen resides at the Upper Dan Tian (the third eye).

Shen, Cun-Zhong 沈存中
One of two authors of the book, *Su Shen Lian Fang (Good Prescriptions of Su and Shen)* The other author is Su, Dong-Po.

Shenque (Co-8) 神闕
An acupuncture cavity belonging to the Conception Vessel.

Shi Er Duan Jin 十二段錦
Twelve Pieces of Brocade. A Qigong set created by Marshal Fei during the Chinese Southern Song dynasty. Later, it was simplified into Ba Duan Jin or Eight Pieces of Brocade.

Shi Er Zhuang 十二庄
Twelve Postures. A Qigong practice created during the Chinese Qing dynasty.

Shi Ji 史紀
Historical Record. A book written in the Spring and Autumn and Warring States Periods (770-221 B.C.).

Shi San Shi 十三勢
Thirteen Postures. An alternative name of Taijiquan.

Shou Jue Yin Xin Bao Luo Jing 手厥陰心包絡經
Arm Absolute Yin Pericardium Channel. One of the twelve primary Qi channels.

Shou Shao Yang San Jiao Jing 手少陽三焦經
Arm Lesser Yang Triple Burner Channel. One of the twelve primary Qi channels.

Shou Shao Yin Xin Jing 手少陰心經
Arm Lesser Yin Heart Channel. One of the twelve primary Qi channels.

Shou Tai Yang Xiao Chang Jing 手太陽小腸經
Arm Greater Yang Small Intestine Channel. One of the twelve primary Qi channels.

Shou Tai Yin Fei Jing 手太陰肺經
Arm Greater Yin Lung Channel. One of the twelve primary Qi channels.

Shou Yang Ming Da Chang Jing 手陽明大腸經
Arm Yang Brightness Large Intestine Channel. One of the twelve primary Qi channels.

Shui 水
Water.

Si Xin Hu Xi 四心呼吸
Four Gates Breathing. A Qigong breathing technique in which the Qi is led to exit or enter the four gates in the center of palms and soles.

Si 四
One of the six healing sounds which regulates the imbalance of Qi in the lungs.

Si 嘶
The sound that is used to help keep warm, in combination with keeping the limbs close to the body and breathing deeply.

Sichuan Province 四川省
A province in western China.

Song dynasty 宋朝
A dynasty in Chinese history (960-1279 A.D.).

Song Gang 鬆肛
Relax the Anus. One of the tricks used to release Qi outside of the body, in coordination with the breathing.

Song Mountain 嵩山
A mountain located in Deng Feng Xian of Henan Province, where the Shaolin Temple is located.

Southern Song dynasty 南宋
After the Song was conquered by the Jin race from Mongolia, the Song people moved to the south and established another country, called Southern Song (1127-1280 A.D.).

Su, Dong-Po 蘇東坡
One of the most famous poets of the Chinese Tang dynasty (618-907 A.D.). Su, Dong-Po was the co-author with Shen, Cun-Zhong of *Su Shen Lian Fang (Good Prescriptions of Su and Shen)*.

Su Wen 素問
The name of a medical book. The complete name of the book is called *Huang Di Nei Jing Su Wen (The Yellow Emperor's Classic)*. This book was written by Ling Shu during the Chinese Han dynasty (circa 100-300 B.C.).

Suan Ming Shi 算命師
Literally, "Calculate Life Teacher." A fortune teller who can calculate your future and destiny.

Sui dynasty 隋
A dynasty in China from 581-618 A.D.

Suliao (Gv-25) 素髎
An acupuncture cavity on the Governing Vessel.

Sun, Si-Mao 孫思邈
A well known Chinese physician and Qigong master who wrote the book, *Qian Jin Fang (Thousand Gold Prescriptions)* between the Sui and Tang dynasties (581-907 A.D.).

Tai Shang Yu Zhou Zhen Jing 太上玉軸眞經
A Daoist classic which records the six healing sounds.

Tai Xi Jing 胎息經
Classic of Harmonized Embryonic Breathing. An important text about embryo breathing in Nei Dan practice.

Taiji (Tai Chi) 太極
Means "Grand Ultimate." It is this force which generates two poles, Yin and Yang.

Taijiquan (Tai Chi Chuan) 太極拳
A Chinese internal martial style based on the theory of Taiji (Grand Ultimate).

Taipei 台北
The capital city of Taiwan.

Taiwan 台灣
An island to the south-east of mainland China. Also known as Formosa.

Taiwan University 台灣大學
A well known university in northern Taiwan.

Taiyang 太陽
Extreme Yang. A very strong and young Yang state.

Taiyang martial stylists 太陽宗
A school of Chinese martial arts that practices Huo Long Gong (Fire Dragon Gong) Qigong training.

Taiyin 太陰
Extreme Yin. A very strong and young Yin state.

Taizuquan 太祖拳
A style of Chinese external martial arts.

Tang dynasty 唐朝
A dynasty in Chinese history from 618-907 A.D.

Tamkang 淡江
A university in Taiwan.

Tamkang College Guoshu Club 淡江國術社
A Chinese martial arts club founded by Dr. Yang when he was studying at Tamkang College.

Tao, Hong-Jing 陶弘景
A well known physician and Qigong master who compiled the book, *Yang Shen Yan Ming Lu (Records of Nourishing the Body and Extending Life)* between 420 to 581 A.D.

Ti 提
Lift.

Ti Xi 體息
Body Breathing. Also called Skin Breathing.

Tian Chi 天池
Heaven's Pond. The place under the tongue that generates saliva during meditation.

Tian Tai Zong 天台宗
Heaven Platform Style. A Qigong style.

Tian Shi 天時
Heavenly Timing. The repeated natural cycles generated by the heavens such as: seasons, months, days and hours.

Tianlinggai 天靈蓋
Heaven Spiritual Cover. A location on the crown of the head.

Tianzong (SI-11) 天宗
An acupuncture cavity on the small intestine primary Qi channel.

Tie Ban Qiao 鐵板橋
Literally, "Iron Board Bridge." Martial arts strength and endurance training for the torso.

Tie Bu Shan 鐵布衫
Iron Shirt. Gongfu training which toughens the body externally and internally.

Tie Sha Zhang 鐵砂掌
Literally, "Iron Sand Palm." Special martial arts conditioning for the palms.

Tong Zi Bai Fo 童子拜佛
The Child Worships the Buddha. A Qigong posture.

Tu 土
Earth.

Tui Na 推拿
Means "To Push and Grab." A category of Chinese massage for healing and injury treatment.

Tuo Tian 托天
Holding up the Sky. A Qigong posture.

Wai Dan 外丹
Literally "External Elixir." External Qigong exercises in which a practitioner builds up the Qi in the limbs and then leads it to the center of the body for nourishment.

Wai Tai Mi Yao 外台祕要
The Extra Important Secret. A Chinese medical book written by Wang Tao between the Sui and Tang dynasties (581-907 A.D.). This book discusses the use of breathing and herbal therapies for disorders of Qi circulation.

Wai Xiang 外象
External appearance.

Wai Xiang Jie Pou 外象解剖
External Appearance Dissection or Analysis. A way to understand the human body by dissection or by acting physically on the body and observing the results, as in modern laboratory experiments.

Wang Tao 王燾
A well known Chinese physician and Qigong master who wrote the book *Wai Tai Mi Yao (The Extra Important Secret)* between the Sui and Tang dynasties (581-907 A.D.).

Wang Zhen 望診
Looking. A diagnostic technique used in Chinese medicine.

Wang, Fan-An 汪汎庵
A well known Chinese physician who wrote the book *Yi Fan Ji Jie (The Total Introduction to Medical Prescriptions)* during the Qing dynasty.

Wang, Wei-Yi 王唯一
A well known Chinese physician who wrote the book, *Tong Ren Yu Xue Zhen Jiu Tu (Illustration of the Brass Man Acupuncture and Moxibustion)* during the Song dynasty.

Wang, Zu-Yuan 王祖源
A well known Chinese physician who wrote the book, *Nei Gong Tu Shuo (Illustrated Explanation of Nei Gong)* during the Qing dynasty.

Wanmai 腕脈

The martial arts name of a cavity on the inner side of the forearm near the wrist. It is called Neiguan (P-6) in acupuncture.

Wei, Bo-Yang 魏伯陽

A well known physician who wrote the book, *Zhou Yi Can Tong Qi (A Comparative Study of the Zhou (dynasty) Book of Changes)* between the Qin and Han dynasties (221 B.C.-220 A.D.).

Weilu 尾閭

Tailbone.

Wen An district 文安

A county located in Hebei Province.

Wen Zhen 問診

Asking. A diagnostic technique used in Chinese medicine.

Wen Zhen 聞診

Listening and Smelling. Two of the diagnostic techniques used in Chinese medicine.

Western Jin dynasty 西晉

A dynasty in Chinese history (265-317 A.D.).

Wilson Chen 陳威伸

Dr. Yang, Jwing-Ming's friend.

Wu Qin Shi 五禽戲

Five Animal Sports. A set of medical Qigong exercises created by Jun Qing during the Chinese Jin dynasty (265-420 A.D.).

Wu Xing Quan 五形拳

Five Animal Fists. The five animals are the tiger, the leopard, the dragon, the snake, and the crane.

Wu, Jian-Quan 吳鑑泉

The creator of Wu Style Taijiquan.

Wu, Quan-You 吳全佑

Father of Wu, Jian-Quan.

Wudang Mountain 武當山

A mountain in Fubei Province, China.

Wushu 武術

Literally, "Martial Techniques." A common name for the Chinese martial arts. Many other terms are used, including: Wuyi (martial arts), Wugong (martial Gongfu), Guoshu (national techniques), and Gongfu (energy-time). Because Wushu has been modified in mainland China over the past forty years into gymnastic martial performance, many traditional Chinese martial artist have given up this name in order to avoid confusing modern Wushu with traditional Wushu. Recently, mainland China has attempted to bring modern Wushu back toward its traditional training and practice.

Xi 嘻

One of the six healing sounds. It regulates the imbalance of Qi in the Triple Burner.

Xi Sui Jing 洗髓經

Literally, *Washing Marrow/Brain Classic,* usually translated *Marrow/Brain Washing Classic.* A Qigong practice that specializes in leading Qi to the bone marrow to cleanse it, or to the brain to nourish the spirit for enlightenment. It is believed that Xi Sui Jing training is the key to longevity and spiritual enlightenment.

Xia Ceng Qi 下層氣
Lower Level Qi. It implies the Qi or bioelectricity which can be accumulated at the lower Dan Tian through correct breathing techniques.

Xia Dan Tian 下丹田
Lower Dan Tian. Located in the lower abdomen, it is believed to be the residence of water Qi (Original Qi).

Xia Yin 下陰
Groin.

Xiao Ang 蕭昂
Governor of Canton during the Chinese Liang dynasty.

Xiao Sheng 小乘
Hinayana, the Lesser Conveyance, which is generally practiced by ascetic monks and aims for the personal achievement of enlightenment.

Xiao Zhi Guan 小止觀
A Buddhist classic which records the six healing sounds.

Xiao Zhou Tian 小周天
Literally, "Small Heavenly Cycle." Also called "Small Circulation". A Qigong practice in which the mind leads the Qi through the Conception and Governing Vessels.

Xie Qi 邪氣
Evil Qi.

Xing 形
Shape.

Xing Gong 行功
Gongfu of transporting the Qi.

Xing Qi 行氣
Circulating or transporting the Qi.

Xingyi 形意
Shape-Mind. An abbreviation of Xingyiquan.

Xingyiquan (Hsing Yi Chuan) 形意拳
Literally, "Shape-Mind Fist." An internal style of Gongfu in which the mind or thinking determines the shape or movement of the body. Marshal Yue Fei is credited with the creation of the style.

Xinkan 心坎
Sternum. Xinkan is the martial name of the sternum. It is called Jiuwei (Co-15) in acupuncture.

Xinzhu Xian 新竹縣
Birthplace of Dr. Yang, Jwing-Ming in Taiwan.

Xiu Qi 修氣
Cultivate the Qi. "Cultivate" implies to protect, maintain and refine. A Buddhist Qigong training.

Xu 噓
The sound "Xu" is believed to help stop bleeding and calm the liver. The relaxation of the liver in turn relieves pain. Xu is one of the six healing sounds.

Xue 穴
Cavities.

Yang 陽

In Chinese philosophy, the active, positive, masculine polarity. In Chinese medicine, Yang means excessive, overactive, overheated. The Yang (or outer) organs are the Gall Bladder, Small Intestine, Large Intestine, Stomach, Bladder, and Triple Burner.

Yang Jing 陽經

Yang primary Qi channels.

Yang Qi 養氣

Cultivating Qi.

Yang, Ban-Hou 楊班侯

A famous Yang Style Taijiquan master (1837-1890 A.D.) who lived during the Qing dynasty.

Yang, Cheng-Fu 楊澄甫

A famous Yang Style Taijiquan master (1883-1935 A.D.) at the beginning of this century.

Yang, Lu-Shan 楊露禪

The creator of Yang Style Taijiquan (1780-1873 A.D.).

Yang Shen Fu Yu 養生膚語

Brief Introduction to Nourishing the Body. A book written by Chen, Ji-Ru during the Qing dynasty.

Yang Shen Jue 養生訣

Life Nourishing Secrets. A medical book written by Zhang, An-Dao between the Song, Jin, and Yuan dynasties (960-1368 A.D.).

Yang Shen Yan Ming Lu 養身延命錄

Records of Nourishing the Body and Extending Life. A Chinese medical book written by Dao, Hong-Jing between 420 and 581 A.D.

Yang, Jwing-Ming 楊俊敏

Author of this book.

Yangming 陽明

Yang Brightness.

Yasai 牙腮

Cheek. A striking zone in the martial arts. It is called Jiache (S-6) in acupuncture.

Yi 意

Mind. Specifically, the mind that is generated by clear thinking and judgment, and which makes one calm, peaceful, and wise.

Yi Fan Ji Jie 醫方集介

The Total Introduction to Medical Prescriptions. A Chinese medical book written by Wang, Fan-An during the Qing dynasty.

Yi Jin Jing 易筋經

Literally, *Changing Muscle/Tendon Classic,* usually called *The Muscle/Tendon Changing Classic.* Credited to Da Mo around 550 A.D., this work discusses Wai Dan Qigong training for strengthening the physical body.

Yi Jing 易經

Book of Changes. A book of divination written during the Zhou dynasty (1122-255 B.C.).

Yi Shou Dan Tian 意守丹田

Keep your Yi on your Lower Dan Tian. In Qigong training, the mind concentrates on the Lower Dan Tian in order to build up Qi. After a practitioner circulates Qi, the Qi is always lead back to the Lower Dan Tian before stopping the exercise.

Yin 陰

In Chinese philosophy, the passive, negative, feminine polarity. In Chinese medicine, Yin means deficient. The Yin (internal) organs are the Heart, Lungs, Liver, Kidneys, Spleen, and Pericardium.

Yin Jing 陰經

Yin Primary Qi Channel.

Yingchuang (S-16) 膺窗

An acupuncture cavity on the Stomach Primary Qi Channel.

Yongquan (K-1) 湧泉

Bubbling Well. An acupuncture cavity on the Kidney Primary Qi Channel.

Yue Fei 岳飛

A Chinese hero from the Southern Song dynasty (1127-1279 A.D.). Fei is said to have created Ba Duan Jin, Xingyiquan and Yue's Ying Zhua.

Yun Gong 運功

Gongfu of transporting the Qi.

Yun Qi 運氣

Transporting the Qi.

Yuzhen 玉枕

Jade Pillow. One of the three gates in Small Circulation meditation.

Zen (Chan) 忍(禪)

Means " To endure." The Japanese name of Chan.

Zhang, An-Dao 張安道

A well known Chinese physician and Qigong master who wrote the book, *Yang Shen Jue (Life Nourishing Secrets),* between the Song, Jin, and Yuan dynasties (960-1368 A.D.).

Zhang, San-Feng 張三豐

Zhang, San-Feng is credited with the creation of Taijiquan during the Song dynasty in China (960-1127 A.D.).

Zhang, Xiang-San 張詳三

A well known Chinese martial artist in Taiwan.

Zhang, Zhong-Jing 張仲景

A well known Chinese physician who wrote the book, *Jin Kui Yao Lue (Prescriptions from the Golden Chamber),* between the Qin and Han dynasties (221 B.C.-220 A.D.).

Zhang, Zi-He 張子和

A well known Chinese physician who wrote the book, *Ru Men Shi Shi (The Confucian Point of View),* between the Song, Jin, and Yuan dynasties (960-1368 A.D.).

Zheng Hu Xi 正呼吸

Formal Breathing. More commonly called Buddhist Breathing.

Zheng Qi 正氣

Righteous Qi. When a person is righteous, it is said that he or she has righteous Qi which evil Qi cannot overcome.

Zhi Zhe Da Shi 智者大師

A Buddhist monk of the Tian Tai branch who wrote the text of *Xiao Zhi Guan.*

Zhong Nan Mountain 終南山

A mountain located in Shanxi Province, China.

Zhong Sheng 中乘

Praktika, the Middle Way, which is the Buddhism of action, and is mostly practiced by wandering preachers.

Zhong Xian 鐘縣

The county where Wudang Mountain is located in Hubei Province, China

Zhou dynasty 周朝

A dynasty in China from 1122-934 B.C.

Zhou Yi Can Tong Qi 周易參同契

A Comparative Study of the Zhou (dynasty) Book of Changes. A medical and Qigong book written by Wei, Bo-Yang between the Qin and Han dynasties (221 B.C.-220 A.D.).

Zhu Bing Yuan Hou Lun 諸病源候論

Thesis on the Origins and Symptoms of Various Diseases. A Chinese medical book written by Chao, Yuan-Fang between the Sui and Tang dynasties (581-907 A.D.).

Zhu, Dan-Xi 朱丹溪

A well known Chinese physician who wrote the book, *Ge Zhi Yu Lun (A Further Thesis of Complete Study),* between the Song, Jin, and Yuan dynasties (960-1368 A.D.).

Zhuang Zhou 莊周

A contemporary of Mencius who advocated Daoism.

Zhuang Zi 莊子

Zhuang Zhou. A contemporary of Mencius who advocated Daoism. Zhuang Zi also means "the works of Zhuang Zhou." He is the author of *Nan Hua Jing.*

Zou Huo 走火

Fire Deviation. It means the Qi is led to the wrong path.

Zu Jue Yin Gan Jing 足厥陰肝經

Leg Absolute Yin Liver Channel. One of the twelve primary Qi channels.

Zu Shao Yang Dan Jing 足少陽膽經

Leg Lesser Yang Gall Bladder Channel. One of the twelve primary Qi channels.

Zu Shao Yin Shen Jing 足少陰腎經

Leg Lesser Yin Kidney Channel. One of the twelve primary Qi channels.

Zu Tai Yang Pang Guang Jing 足太陽膀胱經

Leg Greater Yang Bladder Channel. One of the twelve primary Qi channels.

Zu Tai Yin Pi Jing 足太陰脾經

Leg Greater Yin Spleen Channel. One of the twelve primary Qi channels.

Zu Yang Ming Wei Jing 足陽明胃經

Leg Yang Brightness Stomach Channel. One of the twelve primary Qi channels.

Zuan 鑽

Drill.

Zuo Chan 坐禪

Sitting meditation.

Index

SELECTED BOOKS FROM YMAA

ANCIENT CHINESE WEAPONS	B004R/671
ANALYSIS OF SHAOLIN CHIN NA	B009/041
ARTHRITIS—CHINESE WAY OF HEALING & PREVENTION	B015R/426
BACK PAIN—CHINESE QIGONG FOR HEALING & PREVENTION	B030/515
BAGUAZHANG	B020/300
CHIN NA IN GROUND FIGHTING	B064/663
CHINESE FAST WRESTLING—THE ART OF SAN SHOU KUAI JIAO	B028/493
CHINESE FITNESS—A MIND / BODY APPROACH	B029/37X
CHINESE QIGONG MASSAGE	B016/254
COMPREHENSIVE APPLICATIONS OF SHAOLIN CHIN NA	B021/36X
EIGHT SIMPLE QIGONG EXERCISES FOR HEALTH, 2ND ED.	B010R/523
ESSENCE OF SHAOLIN WHITE CRANE	B025/353
ESSENCE OF TAIJI QIGONG, 2ND ED.	B014R/639
EXPLORING TAI CHI	B065/424
INSIDE TAI CHI	B056/108
LIUHEBAFA FIVE CHARACTER SECRETS	B067/728
MARTIAL WAY AND ITS VIRTUES	B066/698
MUGAI RYU	B061/183
NORTHERN SHAOLIN SWORD, 2ND ED.	B006R/85X
PRINCIPLES OF TRADITIONAL CHINESE MEDICINE	B053/99X
QIGONG FOR HEALTH & MARTIAL ARTS 2ND ED.	B005R/574
QIGONG FOR LIVING	B058/116
QIGONG MEDITATION - EMBRYONIC BREATHING	B068/736
QIGONG, THE SECRET OF YOUTH	B012R/841
ROOT OF CHINESE QIGONG, 2ND ED.	B011R/507
SHIHAN TE—THE BUNKAI OF KATA	B055/884
TAEKWONDO—ANCIENT WISDOM FOR THE MODERN WARRIOR	B049/930
TAEKWONDO—SPIRIT AND PRACTICE	B059/221
TAI CHI BOOK	B032/647
TAI CHI THEORY & MARTIAL POWER, 2ND ED.	B007R/434
TAI CHI CHUAN MARTIAL APPLICATIONS, 2ND ED.	B008R/442
TAI CHI WALKING	B060/23X
TAIJI CHIN NA	B022/378
TAIJI SWORD, CLASSICAL YANG STYLE	B036/744
TAIJIQUAN, CLASSICAL YANG STYLE	B034/68X
TAIJIQUAN THEORY OF DR. YANG, JWING-MING	B063/432
TRADITIONAL CHINESE HEALTH SECRETS	B046/892
WAY OF KENDO AND KENJITSU	B069/0029
WOMAN'S QIGONG GUIDE	B045/833
XINGYIQUAN	B013R/416

SELECTED VIDEOTAPES FROM YMAA

ADVANCED PRACTICAL CHIN NA SERIES	
ANALYSIS OF SHAOLIN CHIN NA	T004/531
ARTHRITIS—THE CHINESE WAY OF HEALING & PREVENTION	T007/558
BACK PAIN—CHINESE QIGONG FOR HEALING & PREVENTION	T028/566
CHIN NA IN DEPTH SERIES—COURSES 1–12	
CHINESE QIGONG MASSAGE SERIES	
COMPREHENSIVE APPLICATIONS OF SHAOLIN CHIN NA 1&2	
DEFEND YOURSELF 1&2	
EMEI BAGUAZHANG SERIES	
EIGHT SIMPLE QIGONG EXERCISES FOR HEALTH 2ND ED.	T005/54X
ESSENCE OF TAIJI QIGONG	T006/238
MUGAI RYU	T050/467
NORTHERN SHAOLIN SWORD SERIES	
SHAOLIN KUNG FU BASIC TRAINING SERIES	
SHAOLIN LONG FIST KUNG FU SERIES	
SHAOLIN WHITE CRANE GONG FU—BASIC TRAINING SERIES	
SIMPLIFIED TAI CHI CHUAN—24 & 48 FORMS	T021/329
TAIJI BALL QIGONG SERIES 1&4	
TAIJI CHIN NA	T016/408
TAIJI PUSHING HANDS SERIES 1–5	
TAIJI SABER	T053/491
TAIJI & SHAOLIN STAFF - FUNDAMENTAL TRAINING - 1	T061/0088
TAIJI SWORD, CLASSICAL YANG STYLE	T031/817
TAIJI YIN & YANG SYMBOL STICKING HANDS SERIES	
TAIJIQUAN, CLASSICAL YANG STYLE	T030/752
WHITE CRANE QIGONG SERIES	
WU STYLE TAIJIQUAN	T023/477
XINGYIQUAN—12 ANIMAL FORM	T020/310
YANG STYLE TAI CHI CHUAN	T001/181

DVDS FROM YMAA

ANALYSIS OF SHAOLIN CHIN NA (DVD)	DVD012/0231
CHIN NA INDEPTH SERIES—COURSES 1-4/5–8/9-12	
EIGHT SIMPLE QIGONG EXERCISES FOR HEALTH (DVD)	DVD008/0037
ESSENCE OF TAIJI QIGONG (DVD)	DVD010/0215
SHAOLIN KUNG FU FUNDAMENTAL TRAINING - 1&2 (DVD)	DVD009/0207
SHAOLIN LONG FIST KUNG FU - BASIC SEQUENCES (DVD)	DVD007/661
SHAOLIN WHITE CRANE GONG FU BASIC TRAINING 1 & 2	DVD006/599
TAIJIQUAN CLASSICAL YANG STYLE (DVD)	DVD002/645
TAIJI SWORD, CLASSICAL YANG STYLE (DVD)	DVD011/0223
WHITE CRANE HARD & SOFT QIGONG (DVD)	DVD003/637

POSTERS FROM YMAA

TAIJIQUAN CLASSICAL YANG STYLE PARTS 1–3

more products available from...

YMAA Publication Center, Inc. 楊氏東方文化出版中心

4354 Washington Street Roslindale, MA 02131
1-800-669-8892 • ymaa@aol.com • www.ymaa.com

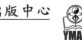